はしがき

　本書は看護英語の総合的な教科書として作成したものです。特に初級の学習者に対して必要な学習内容をConversation, More Expressions, Writing Challenge, Readingといった四技能にまたがる活動にバランスよく含めました。学習者はまず、基本的な会話から始めて、各Unitのテーマに関連した表現、英作文、そして書き下ろしの英文読解へと進むことができます。そして章末のFurther Studyにおいては各Unitのテーマに関連した現代医療における必須の知識やホットトピックを学習することもできます。例えば、近年増加する糖尿病患者の世界分布やバイリンガル登録票、処方せんの様式などを知ることができます。

　本書では、看護の現場で必要な英語の調査に基づき、外国人患者が増加傾向にある現代において実際想定される場面を設定しました。さらに痛み、症状において一般によく使用される語句も精選しました。本書が多くの看護英語学習者の一助にならんことを期待しています。

　本書の出版にあたり金星堂編集部の戸田さんと蔦原さんには根気よく原稿をチェックして頂き、又貴重な御意見を頂きました。厚くお礼を申し上げます。

著者

JN125947

本書の使い方

本書は全15のUnitから成り立ち、以下のように構成されています。

Key Words

Conversationで出てくる重要語句の意味を確認しましょう。

Conversation

A 会話の音声を聞いて、聞き取った英単語を空所に書きましょう。会話は看護師や医師が医療現場で実際に経験しそうな内容になっています。

B イラストの中から、会話の内容に合うものを選びましょう。

C ペアによるロールプレーで、看護師や医師、患者になったつもりで会話に出てきた重要表現を言ってみましょう。

More Expressions

A 会話に出てきた重要表現やプラスアルファの表現をディクテーションで確認しましょう。

B ペアになってAで学んだ表現を声に出して練習しましょう。

Writing Challenge

これまでに学んだ表現や知識を使って英作文にチャレンジしてみましょう。

Reading

120~140語程度の英文読解と内容確認をおこない、医療に関する知識の理解を深めましょう。英文の内容はConversationと共通のテーマになっています。

Further Study

ビジュアル情報とともに、現代医療の知識や話題について楽しく学ぶコーナーです。簡単なクイズもあるので、気軽に挑戦してみましょう。

この他、巻末には付録として医療現場で役立つ重要表現集と人体図を掲載しています。

CHECK-UP!
Basic English for Nursing

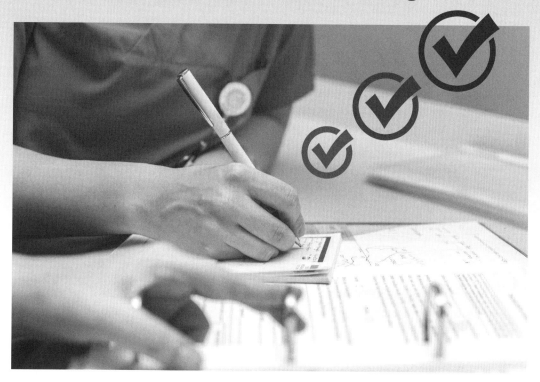

Akihiko Higuchi

John Tremarco

KINSEIDO

Kinseido Publishing Co., Ltd.

3-21 Kanda Jimbo-cho, Chiyoda-ku,
Tokyo 101-0051, Japan

First published 2023 by Kinseido Publishing Co., Ltd.

Cover design   Nampoosha Co., Ltd.
Text design   Asahi Media International Inc.
Illustrations   Miyuki Suzuki

🎧 音声ファイル無料ダウンロード

https://www.kinsei-do.co.jp/download/4184

この教科書で 🎧 DL 00 の表示がある箇所の音声は、上記 URL または QR コードにて無料でダウンロードできます。自習用音声としてご活用ください。

- ▶ PC からのダウンロードをお勧めします。スマートフォンなどでダウンロードされる場合は、ダウンロード前に「解凍アプリ」をインストールしてください。
- ▶ URL は、検索ボックスではなくアドレスバー（URL 表示覧）に入力してください。
- ▶ お使いのネットワーク環境によっては、ダウンロードできない場合があります。

◎ CD 00　左記の表示がある箇所の音声は、教室用 CD（Class Audio CD）に収録されています。

CONTENTS

Unit 1
May I Help You?

UNIT GOAL

□ 初診受付の流れを学ぶ①
□ 症状を伝える基本の表現を学ぶ

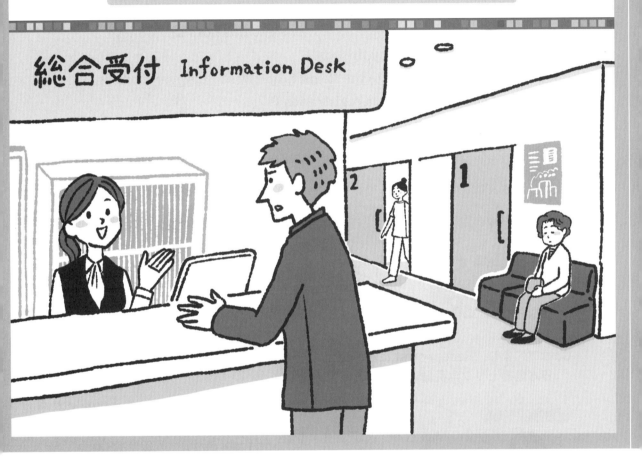

総合受付 Information Desk

Key Words

以下の英語の意味を選択肢から記号で選び、書き入れましょう。

1. receptionist	(	)	**a.**	初めての訪問
2. feel dizzy	(	)	**b.**	受付係
3. first visit	(	)	**c.**	登録カウンター
4. registration desk	(	)	**d.**	目まいがする
5. registration form	(	)	**e.**	登録票

Conversation

A. ハリスさんは初めて訪れた病院のインフォメーションにいます。会話を聞いて空所を埋めましょう。 DL 02　CD 02

● *At the Information Desk*

Receptionist: May I (¹　　　　　　　) you?

Mr. Harris: Yes. I have a fever and I feel dizzy. I (²　　　　　　　) to see a doctor.

Receptionist: Is this your (³　　　　　　　) visit to this hospital?

Mr. Harris: Yes, it is. This is my first visit.

Receptionist: Then, please go to the Registration Desk. It's over there at Window No. 2. You can get a registration (⁴　　　　　　　).

Mr. Harris: OK. I (⁵　　　　　　　). Thank you very much.

Receptionist: Not at all.

B. ハリスさんはこの後何をするでしょう。a～cのイラストから選びましょう。

a
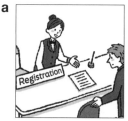

b
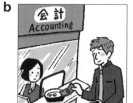

c
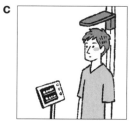

C. ペアになり、Receptionist と Patient になったつもりでロールプレーをしましょう。日本語のセリフは英語に直して言ってみましょう。

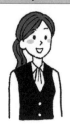

Receptionist

May I help you?

I have a fever and I feel dizzy.

Patient

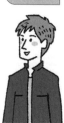

この病院に来るのは初めてですか？

はい、そうです。今回が初めての訪問です。

More Expressions

A. 音声を聞き、日本語に合うように空所を埋めましょう。　 DL 03　CD 03

1. I have a ( ).	熱があります。
2. I feel ( ).	めまいがします。
3. I have ( ) cold.	風邪です。
4. I ( ) nauseous.	吐き気がします。
5. I have the ( ).	寒気がします。
6. I have a ( ) nose.	鼻水が出ています。
7. I have high/low ( ) pressure.	高血圧／低血圧です。
8. I feel ( ).	気分が悪いです。

B. ペアになり、1人はAの日本語を読み上げましょう。もう1人は教科書を閉じ、読み上げられた日本語に対応する英語の表現を言ってみましょう。

 いくつ言えましたか？

☐ 😃 7〜8つ　　☐ 😐 4〜6つ　　☐ 😣 1〜3つ
Excellent　　　　**Average**　　　　**Poor**

Writing Challenge

以下の日本語を英語で書きましょう。

1. 今朝、少しめまいがしました。

I felt _____ .

2. 寒気がします。たぶん風邪をひいています。

_____ . Maybe _____ .

3. 吐き気がしますか。―いいえ。大丈夫です。

Do you _____ ? ―No. _____ .

Reading

英文を読んで以下の問いに答えましょう。

 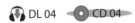

Mr. Harris wasn't feeling well. He was feeling hot and chilly at the same time, and he felt dizzy when he stood up. He had not slept well the night before because

5　he was vomiting throughout the night. After he told his fiancée of his condition,

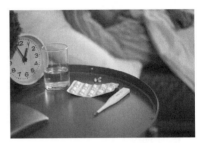

she insisted that she take his temperature. "It's 38 degrees. You have a fever; you should go to the hospital," she told him. He was a little confused on arrival at the hospital because it was his first time. At reception, he was

10　directed to the registration desk to get a registration form. The reception staff was very helpful, but he started to worry because he was thinking about how his condition would affect his ongoing high blood pressure problem.

(126 words)

Notes

insist that... 「～するように主張する、強く言う」　be confused 「困惑する」
direct... 「（動）～を案内する」　affect... 「～に影響する」　ongoing 「進行中の、続いている」

1. Why wasn't Mr. Harris feeling well?

(a) He had been drinking alcohol the night before.

(b) He had a fever, and he felt dizzy when he stood up.

(c) He has low blood pressure.

2. Why didn't Mr. Harris sleep well?

(a) He had been vomiting throughout the night.

(b) He had been drinking alcohol throughout the night.

(c) He had been feeling chilly throughout the night.

3. What did Mr. Harris' fiancée insist on?

   (a) She insisted that he go back to bed.

   (b) She insisted that he drink alcohol.

   (c) She insisted that she should take his temperature.

 登録票／診察申し込み書においては少なくとも以下のような項目を記入する必要があります。以下のフォームの下線部に自分の情報を英語で書いてみましょう。また、(　　)内に適切な日本語を入れてみましょう。

Registration Form / Medical Questionnaire

KSD CLINIC

Name（名前）	Date of Birth（生年月日）※西暦で書く
_____	_____
Sex（性）※□に✓を入れる □ Male（男）　□ Female（女）　□ Other（その他）	Nationality（国籍） _____
Present Address（現住所） _____	Telephone Number（電話番号） _____
What is wrong with you?（　　　　　　　　　　　　　　　　） _____	
How long have you had these problems?（　　　　　　　　　　　） _____	

Unit 2
Where Do You Live?

UNIT GOAL

☐ 初診受付の流れを学ぶ②
☐ 初診登録に必要な表現を学ぶ

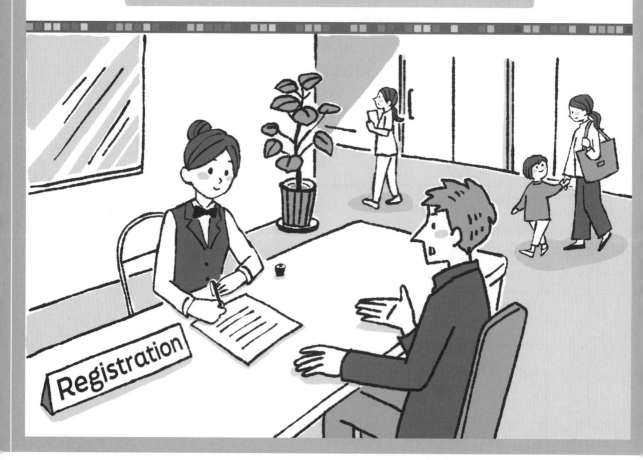

Registration

Key Words

以下の英語の意味を選択肢から記号で選び、書き入れましょう。

1. fill in	( )	**a.** 結婚の有無
2. date of birth	( )	**b.** 記入する
3. marital status	( )	**c.** 現住所
4. single	( )	**d.** 独身の
5. present address	( )	**e.** 生年月日

Conversation

A. ハリスさんは病院で初診登録をします。会話を聞いて空所を埋めましょう。

DL 05　　CD 05

● *At the Registration Desk*

Clerk: Thank you for waiting. This is the registration form you need to
　　(¹　　　　　　) in.

Mr. Harris: Oh, I can't read Japanese.

Clerk: That's OK. I'll help you. May I have your (²　　　　　) and date of
　　birth, please?

Mr. Harris: My name is Harris. James Harris. I was born on November 11, 1990.

Clerk: OK. Mr. Harris. May I ask your (³　　　　　　) status?

Mr. Harris: Sure, I'm single.

Clerk: Uh-huh. (⁴　　　　　) do you live, Mr. Harris?

Mr. Harris: I live in Nerima. My present address is Room 308 Sun City, 2831
　　Koyama, Nerima-ku, Tokyo.

Clerk: All right. Let me (⁵　　　　　) your registration card... Now, your
　　registration card is ready, Mr. Harris.

B. ハリスさんの現在の家族構成を、a〜cのイラストから選びましょう。

a
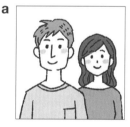
b
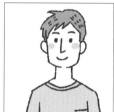
c
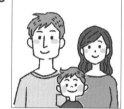

C. ペアになり、Clerk と Patient になったつもりでロールプレーをしましょう。日本語のセリフは英語に直して言ってみましょう。

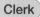 Clerk

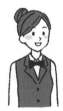

May I have your
name and date of
birth, please?

My name is
(*your name*).
I was born on
(*your birthday/year*).

Patient

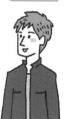

ご結婚されて
いますか。

いいえ、
私は独身です。

Unit 2 Where Do You Live?　　**7**

A. 音声を聞き、空所を埋めましょう。その後、空所に入った語句の意味を考えてみましょう。 🎧 DL 06 💿 CD 06

---

1. My (　　　　　　　　) (　　　　　　　　　) is Building 5, 2010 Minami-ku, Fukuoka City, 815-0071.

2. My (　　　　　　　　) (　　　　　　　　　) is 3777 Nishiyokamachi, Saga City, 840-0036.

3. My (　　　　　　　　) (　　　　　　　　　) is Room 3, 233-3 Aira City, Kagoshima, 899-5492.

英語で日本での住所を書く場合は、日本語とは逆の順番で書きます。したがって、部屋番号、番地を書いてから、市、都道府県と続きます。最後に郵便番号を書きます。アメリカの住所を書く場合、Zip Codeを必ずつけなければなりません。カリフォルニア州ビバリーヒルズの場合はBeverly Hills, CA 90210というように州名の後に表記します。日本での郵便番号に相当するものです。

B. 自分自身の現住所と、学校の住所を英語でそれぞれ書いてみましょう。その後ペアになり、教科書を閉じて学校の住所を英語で言ってみましょう。

自宅の現住所：＿＿＿＿＿＿＿＿＿＿＿＿＿＿＿＿＿＿＿＿＿＿＿＿＿＿＿＿＿＿

学校の住所：＿＿＿＿＿＿＿＿＿＿＿＿＿＿＿＿＿＿＿＿＿＿＿＿＿＿＿＿＿＿＿

 間違えずに言えましたか？

☐ Excellent　　　☐ Average　　　☐ Poor

以下の日本語を英語で書きましょう。

1. この登録票にご記入ください。

Please ＿＿＿＿＿＿＿＿＿＿＿＿＿＿＿＿＿＿＿＿＿＿＿＿＿＿＿＿＿＿＿.

2. 彼の名前はRobert Brownで独身です。

His name ＿＿＿＿＿＿＿＿＿＿＿＿＿＿＿＿＿＿＿＿＿＿＿＿＿＿＿＿＿.

3. 彼の現住所は90210 California州Beverly Hills 684 North Linden Drです。

His present ＿＿＿＿＿＿＿＿＿＿＿＿＿＿＿＿＿＿＿＿＿＿＿＿＿＿＿＿.

Reading

英文を読んで以下の問いに答えましょう。

 DL 07   CD 07

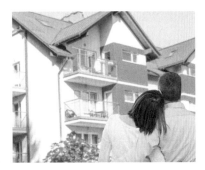

Mr. Harris is a single man living in Nerima. His present address is Room 308 Sun City, 2831 Koyama. However, his marital status is about to change because
5 he is engaged to Akiko Yamashita, a nurse working at Nerima General Hospital. His present address is a tentative one because he and his fiancée hope to move to a new apartment block in Shinjuku in the summer. If all goes well, their Shinjuku apartment will become their
10 permanent home. To make all this happen, Mr. Harris has to go to the town hall on Wednesday to fill in some registration forms. He is worried about this because he cannot read Japanese. Akiko cannot go with him because she has to work every weekday.

(122 words)

Notes

be engaged to...「～と婚約している」   apartment block「アパート（マンション）」
town hall「（市や区の）役所、庁舎」

1. Why is Mr. Harris' marital status about to change?
  (a) He is divorced.
  (b) He is engaged to Akiko Yamashita.
  (c) He is married to Akiko Yamashita.

2. Why is his present address a tentative one?
  (a) He will live there permanently.
  (b) He and his fiancée plan to move to Shinjuku.
  (c) He plans to buy the house that he lives in now.

Unit 2 Where Do You Live?   **9**

3. Why is Mr. Harris worried about filling in the registration forms at the town hall?

    (a) He is very good at reading Japanese.

    (b) He cannot read Japanese.

    (c) The registration forms are very expensive.

Further Study

病院の登録票に記入する必要事項の中には、氏名や住所や生年月日のほか、「婚姻の有無」(marital status) や「緊急連絡先」、かかりつけ医などについて記入する場合もあります。さらに外国人患者向けの登録票には、言語や宗教に関する項目が含まれることもあります。以下のフォームの下線部に自分の情報を英語で書いてみましょう。また、(　　)内に適切な日本語を入れてみましょう。

Registration Form / Medical Questionnaire

KSD CLINIC

Marital status（婚姻の有無）	□Single（独身）　　□Married（既婚）　　□Divorced（離婚） ※□に✓を入れる
Emergency contact （　　　　　　　　　）	Name / Relationship _____ Contact number _____
Family doctor（かかりつけ医）	Doctor's name _____ Contact number _____
Interpreter request（通訳の要請）	□Yes　□No　※□に✓を入れる
Special considerations for religious reasons, etc. （宗教などの理由による配慮）	_____ _____

Unit 3

Do You Have an Insurance Card?

UNIT GOAL

□ 初診受付の流れを学ぶ③
□ 保険に関する表現を学ぶ

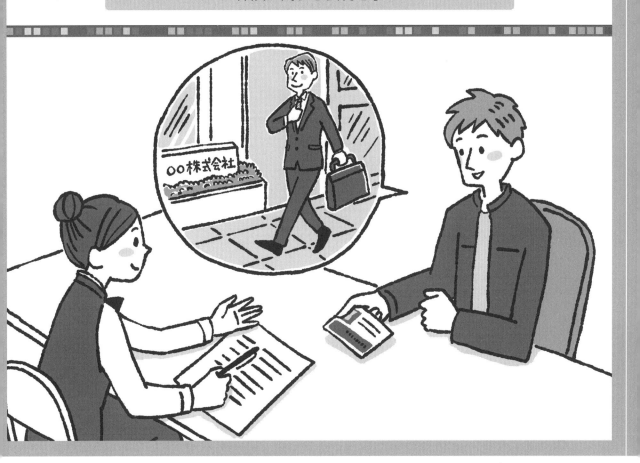

Key Words

以下の英語の意味を選択肢から記号で選び、書き入れましょう。

1. insurance card 　　　（　　　）　**a.** 事務室

2. Japanese company 　（　　　）　**b.** 重要な

3. health insurance card （　　　）　**c.** 保険証

4. office 　　　　　　　（　　　）　**d.** 健康保険証

5. important 　　　　　（　　　）　**e.** 日本の会社

Conversation

A. 登録が終わったハリスさんは次に何をするでしょう。会話を聞いて空所を埋めましょう。

DL 08　　CD 08

● *At the Registration Desk*

Clerk: OK. Your registration card is ready. Do you have an
(**¹**　　　　　　　　) card, Mr. Harris?

Mr. Harris: Oh, yes I do. You mean health insurance, right? I'm
(**²**　　　　　　　　) at a Japanese company and I have my own health
insurance card. Here you are.

Clerk: Good. This is your health insurance card. When you come to the
hospital, you (**³**　　　　　) to show this card to the office. This is an
important thing you need to remember.

Mr. Harris: OK. Is there anything else?

Clerk: No, that's all. Please (**⁴**　　　　　) there. A (**⁵**　　　　　) will call
your name.

Mr. Harris: All right. Thank you very much.

B. 病院を受診するときに必要なものを、a〜cのイラストから選びましょう。

a
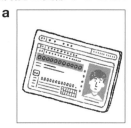

b
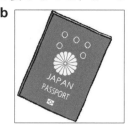

c
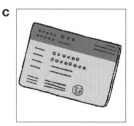

C. ペアになり、Clerk と Patient になったつもりでロールプレーをしましょう。日本語のセリフは英語に直して言ってみましょう。

Clerk

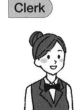

Your registration card is ready.

保険証を持っていますか。

Thank you.

はい、持っています。日本の会社で働いています。

Patient

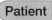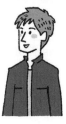

12

More Expressions

A. 音声を聞き、空所を埋めましょう。 DL 09 CD 09

1. What kind of ( ) do you have?
2. I have ( ) insurance.
3. I have ( )-life insurance.
4. My husband works for a ( ) insurance company.
5. Please show me your ( ) Health Insurance Card.

B. 上の英文をヒントに、以下の日本語を英語に直しましょう。その後ペアになり、答えを確認しましょう。

1. 国民健康保険証　（ ）
2. 健康保険　（ ）
3. 損害保険　（ ）
4. 海上保険　（ ）

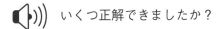 いくつ正解できましたか？

□ 😊 4つ
Excellent

□ 😐 2～3つ
Average

□ 😣 1つ
Poor

Writing Challenge

以下の日本語を英語で書きましょう。

1. 私は日本の会社の健康保険に入っています。

   I have _____ provided by a Japanese company.

2. あなたは損害保険に入っていますか。

   Do you have _____ ?

3. 彼は国民健康保険証を持っていません。

   _____ Insurance Card.

英文を読んで以下の問いに答えましょう。 DL 10 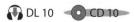 CD 10

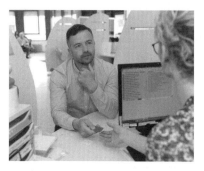

    When a person visits a Japanese hospital, they are required to show their health insurance card. If they do not have a health insurance card,

5 their medical costs will be much higher. This card is called a "hoken-sho" in Japanese. People who work full-time get this card from their employers. People who work part-time can get a health insurance card from their local town hall; this card is called

10 a "Kokumin-Kenko-Hoken-sho" in Japanese. Your health insurance card is very important, so you must remember to take it with you and show it at the reception desk/office when you visit a hospital. If you are required to visit the same hospital again, you will be given a registration card.

(119 words)

Notes

employer「雇用主」　be required to...「～することを求められる」

1. How does a full-time worker get a health insurance card?
- **(a)** They get it from a pharmacy.
- **(b)** They get it from their employer.
- **(c)** They get it from their local town hall.

2. How does a part-time worker get a health insurance card?
- **(a)** They get it from a pharmacy.
- **(b)** They get it from their employer.
- **(c)** They get it from their local town hall.

3. If you are required to visit the same hospital again, what kind of card will you be given?

(a) A pharmacy card

(b) A registration card

(c) A library card

 Further Study 一時的に日本に滞在する外国人旅行客は、医療を受けられるのでしょうか。2019年に行われたある調査によると、約70%の旅行客は何らかの形で旅行保険に加入していましたが、残りの30%弱は「保険の存在を知らなかった」「日本は安全である」などの理由で加入していないことがわかりました。このような状況を踏まえて、近年外国人向け旅行保険のサービスを開始する保険会社が出てきました。これは「インバウンド保険」と呼ばれ、日本入国後でも加入でき、様々な角度から旅行客をサポートしています。

以下はある旅行会社が提供しているインバウンド保険の案内です。（　　）内に適切な語を下の選択肢から選び、書き入れましょう。

Travel Insurance for Visitors
−Stay Safe and Enjoy Your Trip in Japan!−

❀ If you become ill or (¹   ),
we will refer you to a
(²   ) hospital.

❀ If the medical staff doesn't understand your
language, we will arrange for an (³   ).

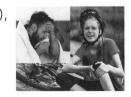

❀ You can pay your medical costs on a
(⁴   ) basis.

interpreter   cashless   suitable   injured

Unit 4
What Department Do You Want to Visit?

UNIT GOAL

- ☐ 患者を案内する
- ☐ 各診療科の名称を学ぶ

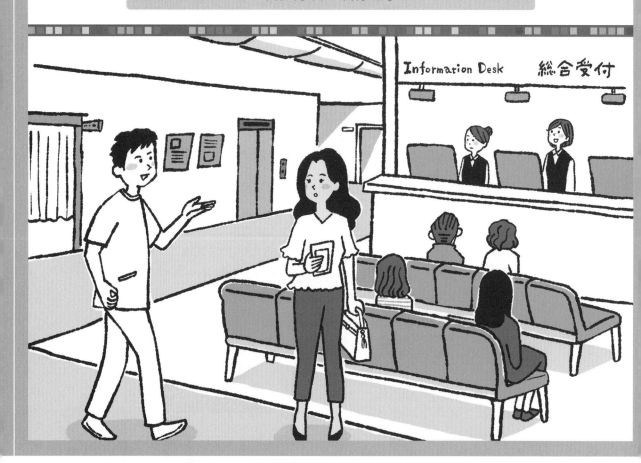

Key Words

以下の英語の意味を選択肢から記号で選び、書き入れましょう。

1. department	(　　)	**a.** 風邪
2. Internal Medicine	(　　)	**b.** 2階
3. cold	(　　)	**c.** 内科
4. second floor	(　　)	**d.** 皮膚科
5. Dermatology	(　　)	**e.** 部局、〜科

Conversation

A. ロペスさんは病院の待合室にいます。会話を聞いて空所を埋めましょう。

DL 11　CD 11

● *At the Information Desk*

Nurse: Hello. What (¹   ) do you want to visit?

Ms. López: I want to visit Internal Medicine because I have a (²   ).

Nurse: All right. It is on the second floor (³   ) to Dermatology.

Ms. López: Where is the elevator?

Nurse: Right over there. I'll show you the way. Be (⁴   ) to bring
your registration card and your insurance card with you.

Ms. López: All right. I'll (⁵   ) you.

B. ロペスさんは次に何をするでしょうか。a〜cのイラストから選びましょう。

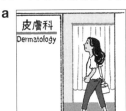 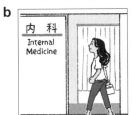 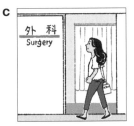

a　皮膚科 Dermatology　　b　内科 Internal Medicine　　c　外科 Surgery

C. ペアになり、Nurse と Patient になったつもりでロールプレーをしましょう。日本
語のセリフは英語に直して言ってみましょう。

Nurse

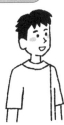

What department
do you
want to visit?

I want to visit
Internal Medicine.

Patient

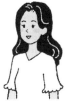

わかりました。
内科は
3階にありますよ。

エレベーターは
どこですか？

More Expressions

A. 音声を聞き、繰り返して発音してみましょう。　DL 12　CD 12

1.	Dermatology	皮膚科
2.	Internal Medicine	内科
3.	Psychiatry	精神科
4.	Pediatrics	小児科
5.	Radiology	放射線科
6.	Cardiology	心臓内科
7.	Surgery	外科
8.	Rehabilitation Services	リハビリテーション部

B. ペアになり、1人はAの日本語を読み上げましょう。もう1人は教科書を閉じ、読み上げられた日本語に対応する英語の表現を言ってみましょう。

 いくつ言えましたか？

☐ 7〜8つ　　☐ 4〜6つ　　☐ 1〜3つ
Excellent　　　　　　**Average**　　　　　　**Poor**

Writing Challenge

以下の日本語を英語で書きましょう。

1. 皮膚科はどこにありますか。

Where _____?

2. 風邪をひいていると思うので、内科に行きたいです。

I think I have a cold, so _____.

3. 保険証と登録カードを必ず持参して下さい。

Be _____ with you.

英文を読んで以下の問いに答えましょう。 DL 13 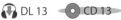 CD 13

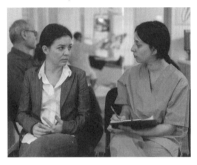

When a patient visits a hospital, they are likely to be asked to wait in the waiting room. It is here that a member of the hospital administration staff, usually
5　a receptionist or a nurse, will ask the patient about their medical problem, and then they will tell the doctor about the condition of the patient. The department a patient will want to visit will very much depend on the medical problem they are suffering from. For
10　example, a patient with a heart condition will want to go to Cardiology. A patient requiring an x-ray will want to go to Radiology. A person suffering from a cold will want to visit the Internal Medicine department. Patients who have skin complaints will want to visit Dermatology.　(125 words)

Notes

be likely to... 「〜するようだ、〜することが多い」　administration staff 「運営スタッフ」
depend on... 「〜次第である」　complaint 「症状、疾患」

1. In the waiting room, who will ask the patient about their medical problem?

　(a) A cardiologist/dermatologist

　(b) A receptionist/nurse

　(c) A radiographer/dermatologist

2. Which department would a patient suffering from a heart condition want to visit?

　(a) Radiology

　(b) Internal Medicine

　(c) Cardiology

3. Which department would a patient suffering from a cold want to visit?

   (a) Cardiology

   (b) Internal Medicine

   (c) Dermatology

総合病院は様々な部局からなり、フロアの面積も広大です。各病院では来院者が目的地にスムーズにたどり着けるように、フロアマップが用意されています。

以下のマップはある病院の１Ｆを示した図です。下の１～３の場合、図中のどの番号へ行ったら良いか、考えてみましょう。

Cherry Blossom Hospital Floor Map

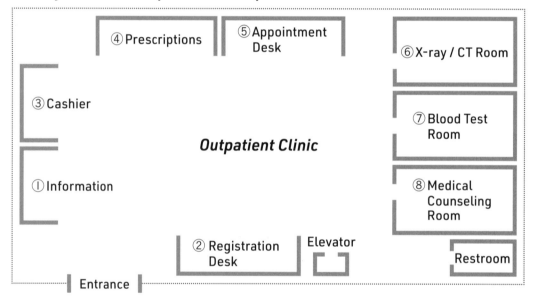

1. 初めての来院時　（　　）

2. Ｘ線検査を受けたい時　（　　）

3. 次回の予約を取りたい時　（　　）

Unit 5
What Are Your Symptoms?

UNIT GOAL

□ 患者の症状を聞く
□ 風邪症状の表現を学ぶ

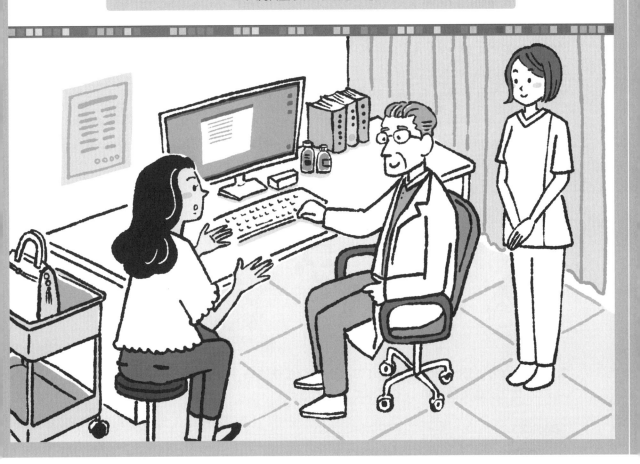

Key Words

以下の英語の意味を選択肢から記号で選び、書き入れましょう。

1. symptom(s)   (   )   **a.** 体温
2. headache   (   )   **b.** せき（をする）
3. cough   (   )   **c.** 症状
4. temperature   (   )   **d.** 頭痛
5. fever   (   )   **e.** 熱

Conversation

A. ロペスさんは診察室に入りました。会話を聞いて空所を埋めましょう。

🎧 DL 14　💿 CD 14

● *In the Doctor's Office*

Doctor: What are your symptoms, Ms. López?

Ms. López: Well, I have a (¹   ) and I have a cough.

Doctor: How long have you been (²   )?

Ms. López: For two days, I guess.

Doctor: Did you check your (³   )?

Ms. López: Yes, I did. It was 38 degrees Celsius this morning.

Doctor: Let's check your temperature (⁴   )... Oh, it's 38.5 degrees now. You have a fever. If you like, we are able to (⁵   ) you a COVID-19 PCR test.

B. ロペスさんの主な症状を、a〜c のイラストから選びましょう。

a 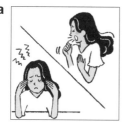　b 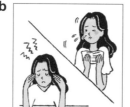　c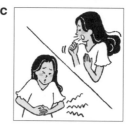

C. ペアになり、Doctor と Patient になったつもりでロールプレーをしましょう。日本語のセリフは英語に直して言ってみましょう。

Doctor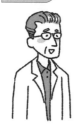

What are your symptoms?

I have a cough.

Patient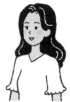

どのくらいの間、せきが続いていますか。

４日間ぐらいだと思います。

More Expressions

A. 音声を聞き、日本語に合うように空所を埋めましょう。 DL 15　CD 15

1. I have a ( ) headache.		ひどい頭痛がします。
2. I ( ) my temperature this morning.		今朝検温しました。
3. I have a ( ) nose.		鼻水が出ています。
4. I feel very ( ).		とても疲れています。
5. I have itchy ( ).		目がかゆいです。
6. Her temperature is 36.5 degrees Celsius.		
It is ( ).		彼女の体温は36.5度です。それは平熱です。
7. My son has a ( ) fever.		私の息子は微熱があります。

B. ペアになり、1人はAの日本語を読み上げましょう。もう1人は教科書を閉じ、読み上げられた日本語に対応する英語の表現を言ってみましょう。

 いくつ言えましたか？

☐ 6〜7つ　　☐ 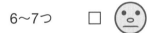 3〜5つ　　☐ 1〜2つ

Excellent　　　　　　**Average**　　　　　　**Poor**

Writing Challenge

以下の日本語を英語で書きましょう。

1. 現在、私は微熱があります。

Currently, _____ fever.

2. あなたの現在の症状は何ですか。

What are _____ ?

3. 私は風邪をひいていてこの3日間ずっとせきをしていました。

_____ for the last three days.

Reading

英文を読んで以下の問いに答えましょう。 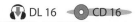 DL 16　CD 16

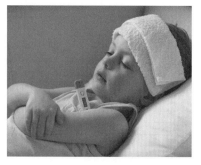

A symptom is something a patient can feel when they are suffering from a medical problem.　One example of a symptom is a fever.　A fever is the body's

5　way of telling us that there is something wrong.　A doctor or nurse can check for a fever by taking a person's temperature.

Most people agree that a temperature of 38 degrees Celsius (100.4 degrees Fahrenheit) is a sign of a fever.　A fever is a symptom, not an illness.　Some

10　common symptoms of COVID-19 include a fever, a dry cough and tiredness. Other less common symptoms include headaches, a sore throat and loss of taste or smell.　Serious symptoms of COVID-19 can include difficulty breathing, chest pain and loss of speech or movement.

(123 words)

Notes

Celsius / Fahrenheit 「摂氏（℃）と華氏（℉）」
※日本では摂氏が一般的に用いられるが、米国をはじめ海外では華氏が用いられる国も多い。
　換算式は以下の通り。摂氏（℃）＝（華氏（℉）−32）÷1.8 ／ 華氏（℉）＝摂氏（℃）×1.8＋32
tiredness 「倦怠感」

1. What is a symptom?

　(a) A symptom is a serious illness.

　(b) A symptom is something a patient can feel when they are suffering from a medical problem.

　(c) A symptom is something a patient feels when they are free from a medical problem.

2. What is a fever?

　(a) A fever is a serious illness.

　(b) A fever is the body's way of telling us that there is something wrong.

　(c) A fever is the body's way of telling us that there is nothing wrong.

3. Which of the following is a serious symptom of COVID-19?

   (a) Difficulty breathing

   (b) A fever

   (c) Headaches

 Further Study 新型コロナウイルス感染症の流行が拡大し始めた当初、インフルエンザや風邪の症状との見分けが難しく、様々な情報がメディアに飛び交いました。以下はある病院が紹介している症状の見分け方の表です。表内の（　）内に、症状名の日本語を書き入れましょう。

Symptom	COVID-19	Flu	Cold
Fever （発熱）	Common	Common	Sometimes
Cough （せき）	Common	Common	Common
Loss of smell/taste (¹)	Common	Sometimes	Sometimes
Shortness of Breath (²)	Sometimes	Rare	Never
Headaches （頭痛）	Common	Common	Sometimes
Muscle aches (³)	Sometimes	Common	Sometimes
Fatigue (⁴)	Common	Common	Sometimes

※この見分け方はあくまで一例です。症状は個々人で異なるため、正確な診断は医師による診察や検査が必要とされます。

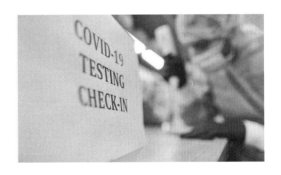

Unit 6
Take One Tablet Three Times a Day

UNIT GOAL

☐ 薬の処方について学ぶ
☐ 服薬指示の表現を学ぶ

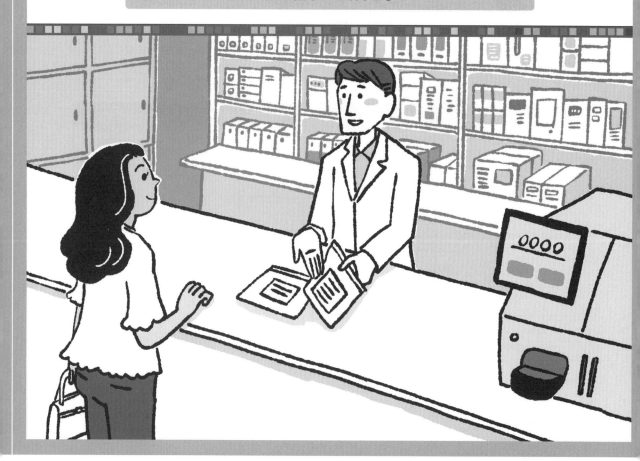

Key Words

以下の英語の意味を選択肢から記号で選び、書き入れましょう。

1. medicine	( )	**a.**	錠剤
2. tablet	( )	**b.**	〜を和らげる
3. antibiotics	( )	**c.**	食事
4. ease	( )	**d.**	抗生物質
5. meal	( )	**e.**	薬

Conversation

A. ロペスさんは薬局にやってきました。会話を聞いて空所を埋めましょう。

DL 17　　CD 17

● *At the Pharmacy*

Pharmacist: Your medicine is (¹　　　　　　　　), Ms. López.

Ms. López: Thank you. What kind of medicine is it?

Pharmacist: These tablets are antibiotics and they help (²　　　　　　　) coughing.

Ms. López: That's good. How often should I (³　　　　　　) them?

Pharmacist: Take one tablet three times after (⁴　　　　　).

Ms. López: With a (⁵　　　　　) of water?

Pharmacist: Yes, exactly.

Ms. López: OK. Thank you very much.

B. ロペスさんが受け取った薬の形状として適切なものを、a〜cのイラストから選びましょう。

a 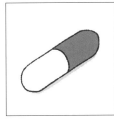　　b 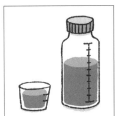　　c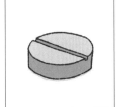

C. ペアになり、Pharmacist と Patient になったつもりでロールプレーをしましょう。日本語のセリフは英語に直して言ってみましょう。

Pharmacist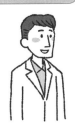

These tablets are antibiotics and they help ease coughing.

How often should I take them?

Patient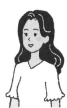

1日3回、1錠を食後に飲んでください。

わかりました。コップ一杯の水で飲みますか。

More Expressions

A. 音声を聞き、空所を埋めましょう。　 DL 18　CD 18

> 1. Take one capsule three times (　　　) (　　　　　　).
> 2. Take this medicine as (　　　　　　).
> 3. Take two tablets (　　　　　　) four hours.
> 4. You can take (　　　　　　) reliever when you have a fever.
> 5. Even after you feel better, you can't (　　　　　) (　　　　　)
>   the antibiotics.

B. 上の英文をヒントに、以下の日本語を英語に直しましょう。その後ペアになり、答えを確認しましょう。

1. 3時間おきに　　　(　　　　　　　　　　　　　　　　　　　　　　　　　)
2. 1日に3回　　　　(　　　　　　　　　　　　　　　　　　　　　　　　　)
3. 必要に応じて　　(　　　　　　　　　　　　　　　　　　　　　　　　　)
4. 抗生物質　　　　(　　　　　　　　　　　　　　　　　　　　　　　　　)
5. 痛み止め　　　　(　　　　　　　　　　　　　　　　　　　　　　　　　)

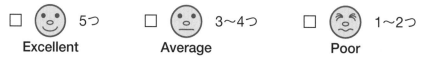 いくつ正解できましたか？

□ 😊 5つ　　　　　□ 😐 3〜4つ　　　　　□ 😖 1〜2つ
　Excellent　　　　　　Average　　　　　　　　Poor

Writing Challenge

以下の日本語を英語で書きましょう。

1. このカプセルを6時間ごとに飲んでください。

   Take _____.

2. グラス一杯の水でこの錠剤を飲んでください。

   _____ a glass of water.

3. 毎朝、これらの抗生物質を飲んでください。

   _____ every morning.

英文を読んで以下の問いに答えましょう。　　　 DL 19　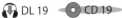 CD 19

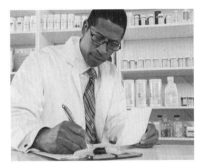

　　　A visit to a hospital often results in a patient being prescribed medicine. Medicine is usually some kind of drug that helps prevent or treat medical

5　problems. It can come in many forms, including tablets, pills, capsules, powders, creams and sprays. For medical problems like colds and flu, tablets are often given to patients to help with pain relief and reducing fever. For bacterial infections, antibiotics are often

10　prescribed. When patients are prescribed medicine, they usually get it from a pharmacy. At the pharmacy, the pharmacist will also give them a medicine/medication regimen. A medicine/medication regimen shows the number or amount of a medicine and the number of times a day the medicine has to be taken or applied.

(121 words)

Notes

prescribe... 「〜を処方する」　relief 「緩和」　bacterial infection 「細菌感染」　apply... 「（薬など）を塗る、つける」

1. Why are patients with colds and flu often given tablets?

(a) They are given tablets to help with pain relief and reducing fever.

(b) They are given tablets to increase their pain and fever.

(c) Many of them have trouble taking powders.

2. Which kind of medicine is given to patients suffering from bacterial infections?

(a) Antihistamines

(b) Creams and sprays

(c) Antibiotics

3. Where do patients usually get their medicines from?

(a) The reception desk

(b) The pharmacy

(c) The nurse station

 調剤薬局で薬を受け取るには、医師が書いた処方せんを提出する必要があります。処方せんには医師の氏名や住所のほか、患者の情報、薬の種類と強さ、服用指示などが記されます。以下の処方せんを見て、下の1〜3の質問に答えましょう。

 Green Leaf Pharmacy
333 Park Ave S, New York, NY 10010
212-555-1111

Patient Name: Adrian Jones
DOB: March 5, 1980
Weight: 176 pounds

R Tussicaps 10mg/8mg caps   Qty. 120
Take 1 cap orally four times daily.
Max 4 caps/day

Refills: 2 refills

Doctor Signature: *Miriam Grace*

Notes

cap「capsuleの略（処方せんには多くの省略記号が用いられる）」
Tussicaps「タッシカプセル（せきやアレルギー由来の上気道症状に処方される）」　max「最多で」

1. この薬はどのような形状ですか。（　　　　　　　　）

2. どのように、1日何回飲みますか。（　　　　　　　　）

3. refill とは何を意味するでしょうか。（　　　　　　　　　　）

Unit 7
You're Suffering from Hay Fever

UNIT GOAL

- ☐ 診察の流れを学ぶ
- ☐ アレルギー症状の表現を学ぶ

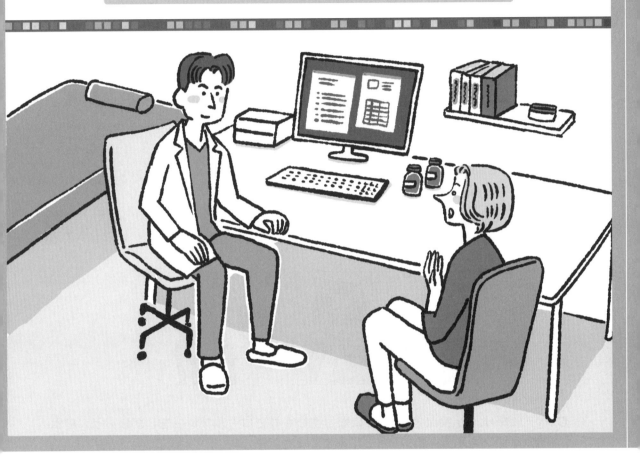

Key Words

以下の英語の意味を選択肢から記号で選び、書き入れましょう。

1. watery （　　） **a.** 涙ぐんだ
2. runny nose （　　） **b.** 花粉症
3. hay fever （　　） **c.** 鼻水
4. pollen （　　） **d.** 抗ヒスタミン
5. antihistamine （　　） **e.** 花粉

Conversation

A. グリーンさんは体調がすぐれず、病院で診察を受けることにしました。会話を聞いて空所を埋めましょう。　🎧 DL 20　💿 CD 20

● *In the Doctor's Office*

Doctor: Good morning, Ms. Green. How are you (¹   ) today?

Ms. Green: I don't feel good today, Doctor. My eyes are itchy and watery. I also have a (²   ) nose.

Doctor: Ah-ha. Do you (³   ) a lot?

Ms. Green: Oh, yes, I do. I sneeze a lot and I also have a stuffy nose.

Doctor: I see. I think you're suffering from hay fever. You are allergic to pollen. We'll (⁴   ) you medicine: antihistamines. These medicines help ease allergy symptoms, such as itchy eyes, sneezing and a stuffy nose.

Ms. Green: That's good! I'm glad to (⁵   ) that. Thank you very much, Doctor.

B. グリーンさんが苦しんでいる症状として<u>当てはまらないもの</u>を、a〜cのイラストから選びましょう。

  a   b   c

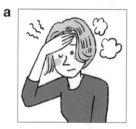 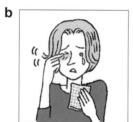 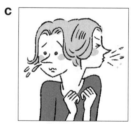

C. ペアになり、Patient と Doctor になったつもりでロールプレーをしましょう。日本語のセリフは英語に直して言ってみましょう。

Patient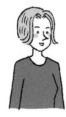

> I have itchy eyes and also have a runny nose.

> Ah-ha. Do you sneeze a lot?

Doctor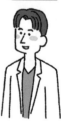

> はい。また、鼻がつまっています。

> あなたは花粉症だと思います。

More Expressions

A. 音声を聞き、空所を埋めましょう。 DL 21　CD 21

> 1. Antihistamines help (　　　　　　　) allergy symptoms.
>
> 2. I have hay fever because I am (　　　　　　) to pollen.
>
> 3. I'm sure you're (　　　　　　) from hay fever.
>
> 4. You're (　　　　　) a lot these days!
>
> 5. I have (　　　　　) eyes almost every day in spring.

B. 上の英文をヒントに、以下の日本語を英語に直しましょう。その後ペアになり、答えを確認しましょう。

1. 目がかゆい　　　　　　　　　(　　　　　　　　　　　　　　　　　)
2. アレルギー症状を緩和する　(　　　　　　　　　　　　　　　　　)
3. 花粉症に苦しむ　　　　　　(　　　　　　　　　　　　　　　　　)
4. たくさんくしゃみをする　　(　　　　　　　　　　　　　　　　　)

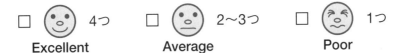
いくつ正解できましたか？

□ 😃 4つ　　□ 😐 2～3つ　　□ 😣 1つ
　Excellent　　　Average　　　　Poor

Writing Challenge

以下の日本語を英語で書きましょう。

1. 私は花粉に対してアレルギーがあります。

_____ pollen.

2. 鼻水が出たり鼻がつまったりします。

　I have _____.

3. 花粉症のため私はくしゃみがたくさん出ます。

　Because of hay fever, _____.

Reading

英文を読んで以下の問いに答えましょう。

 DL 22　CD 22

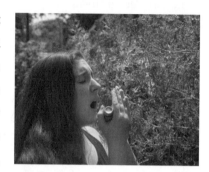

Many people suffer from allergies: according to the UK National Health Service, one in four people suffer from them. An allergy is a condition where
5 the body has a reaction to a food or substance. The substances that cause allergic reactions are called allergens. The most common allergens include dust mites, animal dander and pollen; the allergic reaction to pollen is also known as hay fever. There are people
10 who are allergic to certain foods. Symptoms of an allergic reaction include sneezing, itchy skin, a runny/blocked nose, wheezing and coughing. There are ways to help people manage their allergies. For example, people suffering from food allergies should always read food labels before eating, and people who suffer from hay fever are often prescribed antihistamines
15 to help with their condition.

(130 words)

Notes

National Health Service「(英国) 国民保健サービス (1948年設立の国営医療サービス)」 substance「物質」
dust mite「イエダニ」 animal dander「動物の皮屑 (皮膚や羽などから出る小さな屑)」 wheezing「息切れ」

1. What is an allergy?

　(a) It is a condition where the body has a reaction to a food or substance.

　(b) It is a kind of antihistamine.

　(c) It is a condition where the body needs certain foods or substances.

2. What are the substances that cause allergic reactions in people?

　(a) Antihistamines

　(b) Allergies

　(c) Allergens

3. What are people who suffer from hay fever given to help them with their allergy?

(a) Antioxidants

(b) Antihistamines

(c) Antibiotics

Further Study

花粉症の原因として有名なものはスギやヒノキの花粉ですが、実は一年を通して様々な植物が鼻炎などのアレルギー症状のもととなっています。そのため花粉症は最近では「通年病」とも言われています。

下記は鼻炎などの症状を引き起こす植物についてまとめたものです。1～4の下線部に該当する植物の英語名を選択肢から選んで書き入れましょう。

Common Plants That Trigger Allergies

Spring

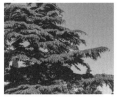

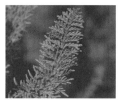

Summer

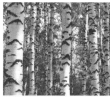

white birch（シラカバ）

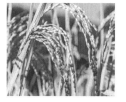

1. _____　（スギ）

2. _____　（ヒノキ）

3. _____　（イネ）

Autumn

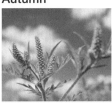

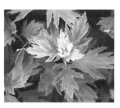

mugwort（ヨモギ）

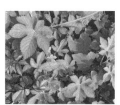

Japanese hop（カナムグラ）

Winter

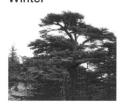

4. _____　（ブタクサ）

1. _____　（スギ）

ragweed	cedar	cypress	rice

Unit 8

What Kind of Pain Is It?

UNIT GOAL

☐ 外科診療の流れを学ぶ
☐ 痛みを表す表現を学ぶ

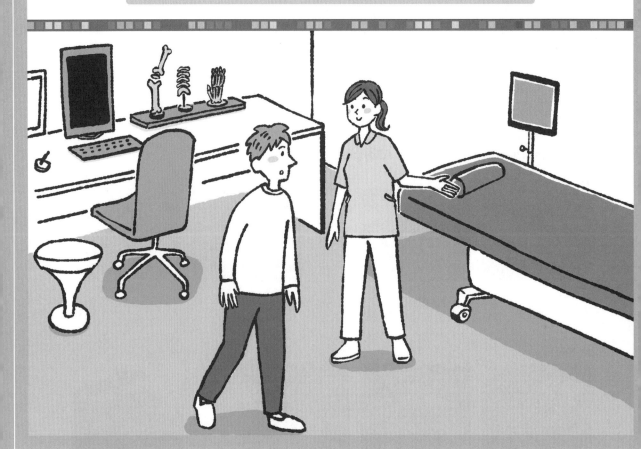

Key Words

以下の英語の意味を選択肢から記号で選び、書き入れましょう。

1. feel pain   (　　)   **a.** 背中

2. back   (　　)   **b.** ひどくなる

3. dull pain   (　　)   **c.** 鈍痛

4. constant   (　　)   **d.** 継続的な

5. get worse   (　　)   **e.** 痛みを感じる

Conversation

A. ハリスさんは整形外科にやってきました。会話を聞いて空所を埋めましょう。

 DL 23　CD 23

● *At Orthopedics*

Nurse: Hello, Mr. Harris. What is your (¹   ) today?

Mr. Harris: I feel (²   ) in my back.　Maybe I hurt my back while

　carrying heavy boxes when I (³   ) last month.

Nurse: What kind of pain is it?

Mr. Harris: It's a (⁴   ) pain and it is constant.

Nurse: Is it getting worse?

Mr. Harris: I (⁵   ) so.

Nurse: Your doctor is coming soon to see you.

B. ハリスさんの問題は何でしょうか。a〜cのイラストから選びましょう。

a 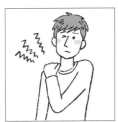　　b 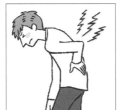　　c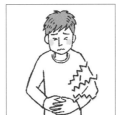

C. ペアになり、Patient と Nurse になったつもりでロールプレーをしましょう。日本語のセリフは英語に直して言ってみましょう。

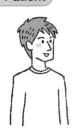

Patient

> I feel pain in my back.

> 鈍い痛みで、ずっと続いています。

Nurse

> What kind of pain is it?

> わかりました。まもなく医師が診察に来ます。

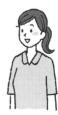

More Expressions

A. 音声を聞き、日本語に合うように空所を埋めましょう。　DL 24　CD 24

1. I have (　　　　　　) pain.	慢性の痛みがあります。
2. I have a (　　　　　).	頭痛がします。
3. It (　　　　　).	ちくちく痛みます。
4. My pain is constant and (　　　　　).	継続的で激しい痛みです。
5. I feel pain in the (　　　　　).	腹部に痛みを感じます。

B. ペアになり、1人はAの日本語を読み上げましょう。もう1人は教科書を閉じ、読み上げられた日本語に対応する英語の表現を言ってみましょう。

 いくつ言えましたか？

☐ ☺ 5つ **Excellent**　　☐ 😐 3〜4つ **Average**　　☐ 😖 1〜2つ **Poor**

Writing Challenge

以下の日本語を英語で書きましょう。

1. 今日はどうなさいましたか。

What is _____?

2. それはどのような痛みですか。

What kind of _____?

3. 私は右肩に痛みを感じます。

_____ right shoulder.

Reading

英文を読んで以下の問いに答えましょう。

 DL 25   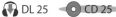 CD 25

Pain is something we are all familiar with because everyone has experienced it at some point in their lives. Pain is often described as an unpleasant physical and/
5 or emotional feeling caused by an injury or illness. There are two major types of pain: chronic and acute. Chronic pain is long, constant pain, and acute pain is short-term pain. It is very difficult to describe pain to a nurse because we cannot "see" it. Hospitals often
10 use numerical pain scales to help patients describe their discomfort. For example, on a 0-10 pain scale, 0 would suggest no pain, 1-3 would suggest mild pain, 4-6 would suggest moderate pain, 7-9 would suggest severe pain, and, finally, 10 would suggest that the pain level is very severe. (125 words)

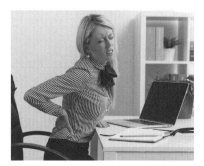

Notes

at some point in one's life「人生のどこかで」　unpleasant「不快な」　acute「急性の」
numerical「数字で表された」

1. Which kind of pain is acute pain?

　(a) It is the kind of pain that lasts a long time.

　(b) It is the kind of pain that lasts a short time.

　(c) It is the kind of pain that causes no unpleasant feeling at all.

2. Why is it difficult for patients to describe pain to a nurse?

　(a) It is difficult because everyone experiences pain at some point in their lives.

　(b) It is difficult because we cannot "see" pain.

　(c) It is difficult because we can easily "see" pain.

3. On a 0-10 numerical pain scale, which level of pain would the number 7 suggest?

(a) It would suggest that the level of pain is mild.

(b) It would suggest that the level of pain is moderate.

(c) It would suggest that the level of pain is severe.

Further Study 英語には痛みを表す表現が数多く存在します。1971年にカナダのマギル大学が開発したMcGill Pain Questionnaireという痛みを評価するためのアンケートには合計78もの痛みを表す単語が掲載されています。radiating pain（放散痛）、tearing pain（裂けるような痛み）など、日本ではあまり使用されないものも含まれます。

日本の医療現場で近年よく用いられているのはPain Scaleという10段階の指標です。10段階の区分はReadingで紹介されていたもののほか、より細かく区分される指標もあります。以下の（　　　　）内に当てはまる痛みの表現を、下の選択肢から記号で選び、書き入れてみましょう。

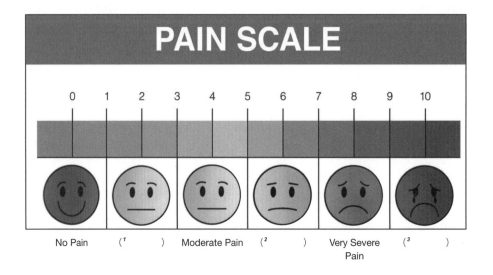

PAIN SCALE

| 0 | 1 | 2 | 3 | 4 | 5 | 6 | 7 | 8 | 9 | 10 |

No Pain　　（¹　　　）　　Moderate Pain　　（²　　　）　　Very Severe Pain　　（³　　　）

a. Worst Pain Possible　　**b.** Mild Pain　　**c.** Severe Pain

Unit 9

Let's Check Your Daily Activities

UNIT GOAL

☐ 問診の流れを学ぶ
☐ 生活習慣を伝える表現を学ぶ

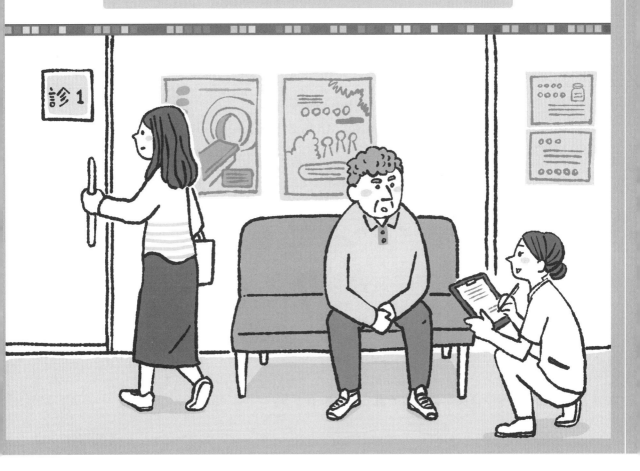

Key Words

以下の英語の意味を選択肢から記号で選び、書き入れましょう。

1. daily activities ( )   **a.** 大酒飲み

2. skip breakfast ( )   **b.** 酒を飲む

3. quit ( )   **c.** 朝食を抜く

4. drink ( )   **d.** やめる

5. heavy drinker ( )   **e.** 生活習慣

Conversation

A. 最近何となく体調の悪いスミスさんは内科を訪れました。会話を聞いて空所を埋めましょう。 DL 26　CD 26

● *At Internal Medicine*

Nurse: Let's check your (¹　　　　　　　) activities, Mr. Smith.

Mr. Smith: OK.

Nurse: Do you eat three meals a day?

Mr. Smith: No, I don't. I sometimes (²　　　　　　) breakfast.

Nurse: Do you smoke?

Mr. Smith: No. I (³　　　　　) ten years ago.

Nurse: That's good for your health, Mr. Smith. How about (⁴　　　　　)?

Mr. Smith: Yes, I do, but I'm not a (⁵　　　　　) drinker.

B. スミスさんが何年も<u>おこなっていないこと</u>を、a〜cのイラストから1つ選びましょう。

 a 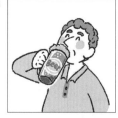 　 b 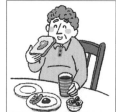 　 c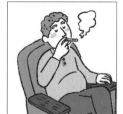

C. ペアになり、NurseとPatientになったつもりでロールプレーをしましょう。日本語のセリフは英語に直して言ってみましょう。

Nurse 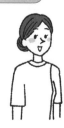　Patient

Let's check your daily activities.

OK.

毎日朝食を食べますか？

いいえ。時々朝食を抜かします。

More Expressions

A. 音声を聞き、空所を埋めましょう。 DL 27 CD 27

> **1.** I drink a (　　　　　) of beer at dinner.
>
> **2.** I eat three (　　　　　) a day.
>
> **3.** I don't (　　　　　). I quit when I got married.
>
> **4.** I sometimes have (　　　　　) between meals.
>
> **5.** Lack of (　　　　　) is bad for your health.

B. 上の英文をヒントに、以下の日本語を英語に直しましょう。その後ペアになり、答えを確認しましょう。

1. 1日3食とる　　　（　　　　　　　　　　　　　　　　　　　　　　）

2. 運動不足　　　　（　　　　　　　　　　　　　　　　　　　　　　）

3. ビール1杯　　　（　　　　　　　　　　　　　　　　　　　　　　）

4. 禁煙する　　　　（　　　　　　　　　　　　　　　　　　　　　　）

5. 軽食をとる　　　（　　　　　　　　　　　　　　　　　　　　　　）

いくつ正解できましたか？

□ ☺ 5つ　　　□ ☺ 3〜4つ　　　□ ☺ 1〜2つ
　Excellent　　　　　Average　　　　　　Poor

Writing Challenge

以下の日本語を英語で書きましょう。

1. 時々食後にタバコを吸います。

I sometimes ＿＿＿＿＿＿＿＿＿＿＿＿＿＿＿＿＿＿＿＿＿ .

2. 酒の飲み過ぎは健康に良くありません。

Drinking too much ＿＿＿＿＿＿＿＿＿＿＿＿＿＿＿＿＿ .

3. 私は朝食にコーヒーとゆで卵 (boiled egg) をとります。

＿＿＿＿＿＿＿＿＿＿＿＿＿＿＿＿＿＿＿ for breakfast.

Reading

英文を読んで以下の問いに答えましょう。

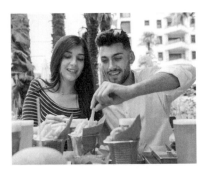

A person's daily activities and routines have a very strong influence on a person's health. Three common activities that have a major negative impact on our health are

5　smoking, drinking alcohol and a poor diet. Smoking can cause cancer, strokes, lung disease and many other health problems. Drinking too much alcohol (heavy drinking) can lead to chronic diseases, high blood pressure, strokes, liver disease and other serious problems. A

10　poor diet can increase stress levels, tiredness and obesity, especially if it is combined with lack of exercise. There is a great deal of debate about the amount of exercise needed to maintain a healthy body, but a lot of medical professionals recommend that adults do at least 150 minutes of moderate activity a week, or 75 minutes of vigorous activity a week. (132 words)

Notes

routine「ルーチン、日課」　stroke「脳卒中、発作」　lung「肺」　liver「肝臓」　obesity「肥満」
be combined with...「～と組み合わさる」　recommend...「～をすすめる」　vigorous「精力的な」

1. What are the effects of a person's daily activities on their health?

　(a) There is a weak connection between a person's activities and their health.

　(b) They have a strong influence on their health.

　(c) They have a strong influence on their wealth.

2. According to the passage, what kind of problems can a poor diet lead to?

　(a) It can increase stress levels, tiredness and obesity.

　(b) It can cause loss of memory.

　(c) It can decrease stress levels, tiredness and obesity.

3. What is the recommended amount of moderate exercise needed to maintain a healthy body?

(a) 150 minutes a week

(b) 75 minutes a week

(c) No exercise at all is needed.

Further Study

生活習慣 (daily activities) についての問診で聞かれることは、食生活、睡眠時間、飲酒、喫煙、薬の服用、薬に対するアレルギーなど細かな内容が含まれます。

例えば食事についてだけでも、以下のような質問をされることがあります。自分自身の食生活を思い起こして、アンケートに答えてみましょう。

Diet Questionnaire

1. Who makes your meals? _____

2. Check all that you do at least twice a week.

☐ Have a late dinner   ☐ Buy pre-prepared meals

☐ Drink sugary drinks   ☐ Eat between meals

☐ Eat greasy food   ☐ Eat out with friends/colleagues

Note
greasy 「油っこい」

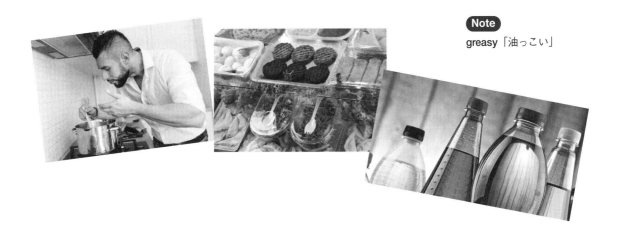

Unit 10
Let's Check Your Pulse and Blood Pressure

UNIT GOAL

□ 診察前の計測をおこなう
□ 計測に関する表現を学ぶ

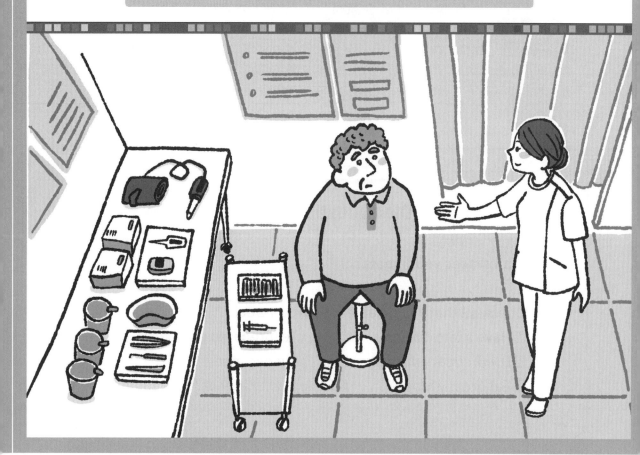

Key Words

以下の英語の意味を選択肢から記号で選び、書き入れましょう。

1. pulse   (   )   **a.** 心配になる

2. get nervous   (   )   **b.** 正常範囲

3. normal range   (   )   **c.** 脈拍

4. high blood pressure (   )   **d.** 高血圧

5. bring... down   (   )   **e.** 〜を下げる、低下させる

Conventsation

A. スミスさんは、医師の診察の前に簡単な健康チェックを受けています。会話を聞いて空所を埋めましょう。 DL 29 CD 29

● *At Internal Medicine*

Nurse: Please have a (¹   ), Mr. Smith. Let's check your pulse and

(²   ) pressure.

Mr. Smith: I'm getting nervous.

Nurse: Don't (³   ), Mr. Smith. Well, your pulse was 70, no

(⁴   ) at all. It was within the normal range.

Mr. Smith: That's good. How about my blood pressure?

Nurse: Let's see. Oh, it's 140 over 80. You have high blood pressure.

Mr. Smith: I can (⁵   ) that because it was also high last year.

Nurse: We should bring it down, Mr. Smith.

B. スミスさんが<u>受けていない</u>検査を、a〜cのイラストから選びましょう。

a 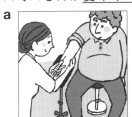　b 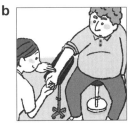　c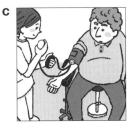

C. ペアになり、Nurse と Patient になったつもりでロールプレーをしましょう。日本語のセリフは英語に直して言ってみましょう。

Nurse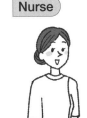

Let's check your pulse and blood pressure.

I'm getting nervous.

Patient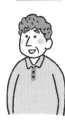

心配しないでください、(*your partner's name*).

ありがとうございます。

More Expressions

A. 音声を聞き、日本語に合うように空所を埋めましょう。 DL 30　CD 30

1. Let's ( ) your weight.		体重を測りましょう。
2. Let's check your ( ).		身長を測りましょう。
3. Let's check your ( ).		脈を測りましょう。
4. Your pulse was within the ( ) range.		
	あなたの脈は正常の範囲内でした。	
5. Your blood pressure is 140 ( ) 82.		
	血圧は上が140、下が82です。	
6. I have a ( ) every year.	毎年健康診断を受けます。	

B. ペアになり、1人はAの日本語を読み上げましょう。もう1人は教科書を閉じ、読み上げられた日本語に対応する英語の表現を言ってみましょう。

🔊)) いくつ言えましたか？

☐ 😃 5～6つ　　☐ 😐 3～4つ　　☐ 😣 1～2つ
Excellent　　　　　Average　　　　　　Poor

Writing Challenge

以下の日本語を英語で書きましょう。

1. あなたの脈拍は正常の範囲内です。

_____ range.

2. あなたの血圧は上が150、下が80です。

_____ .

3. あなたの血圧はとても高いです。下げなくてはなりません。

Your blood pressure _____. We should _____ .

Reading

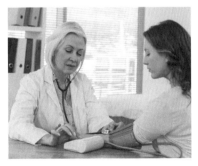

　　When a person goes to a hospital for a check-up, they often feel nervous. Feeling nervous about the check-up is natural, but it should not prevent people from having

5　them on a regular basis. The procedures that a person is likely to undergo during a basic health check usually include taking a person's pulse and blood pressure. A pulse is the number of beats the heart makes in a minute; a normal pulse rate should be between 60 and 100

10　beats per minute. Persistent high blood pressure is a sign that something is wrong with your body. It can increase the risk of several unhealthy conditions that include heart disease, kidney disease and strokes.

(114 words)

Notes

on a regular basis「定期的に」　procedure「工程」　undergo...「〜を受ける、経験する」
persistent「持続的な」　kidney「腎臓」

1. What are two procedures that a person is likely to undergo during a basic health check?
   (a) They will undergo a CAT scan and an MRI scan.
   (b) They will have their pulse and blood pressure taken.
   (c) They will take an IQ test.

2. What is considered to be a normal pulse rate?
   (a) 40 to 70 beats per minute
   (b) 60 to 100 beats per minute
   (c) 100 to 160 beats per minute

3. Which of the following unhealthy conditions can persistent high blood pressure increase the risk of?

(a) Heart disease, kidney disease and strokes

(b) Loss of memory and appetite

(c) Dementia and heart failure

Further Study

一般的な健康診断では体重や身長、視力のほか、血圧も測定されます。私たち人間の血圧の正常な範囲（normal range）は、最高血圧は135 mmHg未満、最低血圧は85 mmHg未満です。高血圧は年齢が上がると発症しやすくなりますが、若者であっても塩分の過剰摂取やストレス、遺伝などの要因で高血圧になることがあるため、注意が必要です。

以下はある学校の健康診断のお知らせです。下の1～3の質問に答えましょう。

Item	Date and Time	Place	What to bring
Chest X-ray	April 2 (Mon)-6 (Fri) 13:30-16:00	Health Support Center	Student ID
Height Weight Eyesight Blood Pressure	April 9 (Mon)-13 (Fri) 9:30-12:30	Student Hall	Student ID
Urinalysis	April 9 (Mon) 9:30-16:00	Health Support Center	Student ID Urine sample

1. 胸部レントゲンと血圧検査は、同じ日に行うことができますか。（　　　　　　）

2. 視力検査と尿検査はそれぞれどこで行われますか。

（　　　　　　　　　　　　　　　）

3. 全ての検査に持っていくべき物は何でしょうか。（　　　　　）

Unit 11

It's Going to Be a Long Day!

UNIT GOAL

- ☐ 患者に検査をすすめる
- ☐ 精密検査に関する表現を学ぶ

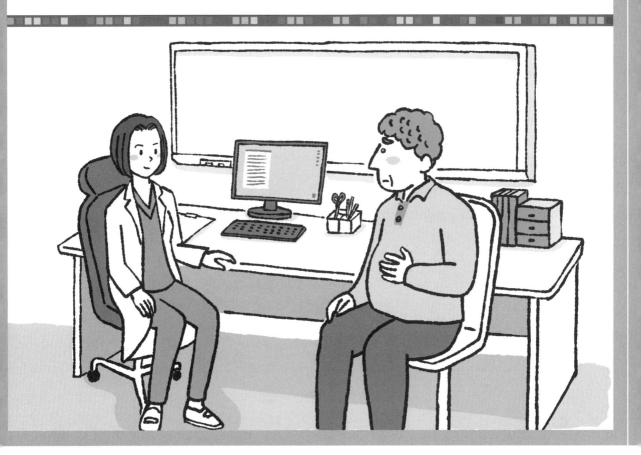

Key Words

以下の英語の意味を選択肢から記号で選び、書き入れましょう。

1. lately   (   )   **a.** 炎症
2. sharp pain   (   )   **b.** 胃カメラ検査
3. stomach   (   )   **c.** 胃、腹部
4. inflammation   (   )   **d.** 最近
5. gastroscopy   (   )   **e.** 鋭い痛み

Conversation

A. スミスさんは、診察室に入り、医師に体調の悩みを相談します。会話を聞いて空所を埋めましょう。　🎧 DL 32　💿 CD 32

● *In the Doctor's Office*

Doctor: Good morning, Mr. Smith. What (¹   ) to be your problem?

Mr. Smith: Well, I don't feel good lately. Sometimes I have sharp pains in my stomach. I'm worried because last year, some inflammations were (²   ) in my stomach.

Doctor: Is that (³   )? Last year you had a gastroscopy. Shall we do it again?

Mr. Smith: When can I take it?

Doctor: How about next Wednesday?

Mr. Smith: (⁴   ) good.

Doctor: That's fine. You'll have a blood test on the (⁵   ) day.

Mr. Smith: Aha, it's going to be a long day!

B. スミスさんが受ける予定の検査を、a〜cのイラストから選びましょう。

a
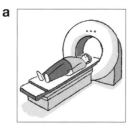

b
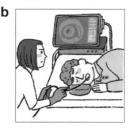

c
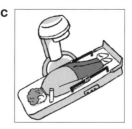

C. ペアになり、DoctorとPatientになったつもりでロールプレーをしましょう。日本語のセリフは英語に直して言ってみましょう。

Doctor
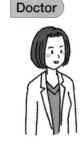

Would you like to take a gastroscopy?

When can I take it?

次の土曜日はどうですか。

良さそうです。

Patient
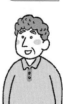

More Expressions

A. 音声を聞き、空所を埋めましょう。

> **1.** I sometimes have sharp pains in my ( ).
>
> **2.** I had a ( ) two years ago.
>
> **3.** Some ( ) were found in my stomach.
>
> **4.** You'll have a ( ) test on the 3rd floor.
>
> **5.** Regular ( ) cancer screening is important.

B. 上の英文をヒントに、以下の日本語を英語に直しましょう。その後ペアになり、答えを確認しましょう。

1. 胃カメラ検査 ( )
2. 血液検査 ( )
3. 炎症を見つける ( )
4. 乳がん検査 ( )

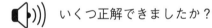 いくつ正解できましたか？

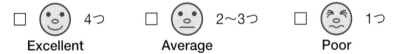

☐ 4つ Excellent   ☐ 2～3つ Average   ☐ 1つ Poor

Writing Challenge

以下の日本語を英語で書きましょう。

1. 私は毎年胃カメラ検査を受けています。

_____ every year.

2. 時々、私は胸に鋭い痛みを感じます。

Sometimes _____.

3. 明日の朝、私は血液検査を受けます。

_____ tomorrow morning.

Reading

英文を読んで以下の問いに答えましょう。　　　　DL 34　　CD 34

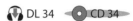

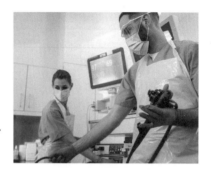

　　In addition to regular medical check-ups, there are occasions when we may have to undergo a more detailed medical examination.　The reasons for such
5　thorough medical examinations usually arise out of concerns over the results of a routine medical examination, or if a patient is exhibiting worrying signs and/or symptoms of a potentially serious medical condition.　The type of procedures undertaken in a
10　thorough examination will depend on the nature of the medical problem a person is suffering from. For example, if there is a problem with a person's stomach, they will undergo a gastroscopy. This is when a thin tube called an endoscope is used to look inside the stomach. Another example of these procedures is the testing for signs of advanced dementia in people over 65.

(128 words)

Notes

thorough「綿密な」　arise out of...「〜から生じる」　exhibit worrying signs「心配な兆候を見せる」
potentially「潜在的に」　endoscope「内視鏡」　dementia「認知症」

1. What is one reason a patient may have to undergo a thorough medical examination?

(a) They don't like regular medical check-ups.

(b) They are showing signs of a potentially serious medical condition.

(c) They are showing signs of a healthy medical condition.

2. What kind of instrument is used in a gastroscopy?

(a) An endoscope

(b) An oscilloscope

(c) A microscope

3. At what age is a person more likely to undergo tests for advanced dementia?

(a) Over 45

(b) Over 55

(c) Over 65

Further Study
上部消化管内視鏡検査（胃カメラ検査）を受ける際、Helicobacter pylori (H. pylori) infection（ピロリ菌に感染しているか否か）について話題になることがあります。ピロリ菌は胃がんや潰瘍の主な原因といわれる厄介な細菌です。日本の感染者は50代、60代が主ですが、世界で見ると2人に1人が感染者であるとも言われています。
ピロリ菌感染症の検査にはいくつかの方法があります。以下ではその中の代表的な3つについて取り上げています。1〜3の検査の具体的な説明にあたるものを選択肢から選びましょう。

1. Breath Test

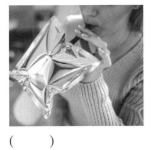

(　　　)

2. Scope Test

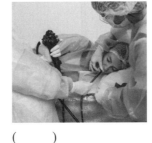

(　　　)

3. Stool Test

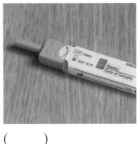

(　　　)

a. It looks for antigens associated with H. pylori infection in your excrement.

b. Samples of exhaled breath will be collected before and after swallowing the test drug.

c. The doctor uses an endoscope to look down into your stomach to take a tissue sample.

Notes
antigen「抗原」　excrement「排泄物」　tissue「組織」

Unit 12
You Have High Blood Sugar Levels

UNIT GOAL

☐ 検査結果を説明する
☐ 数値を伝える表現を学ぶ

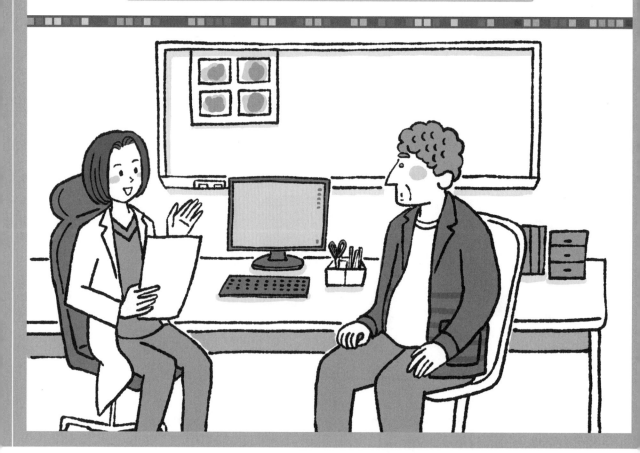

Key Words

以下の英語の意味を選択肢から記号で選び、書き入れましょう。

1. blood test result （　　） **a.** 喉がかわいている
2. blood sugar level （　　） **b.** 血液検査結果
3. value （　　） **c.** 特に
4. feel thirsty （　　） **d.** 血糖値
5. particularly （　　） **e.** 数値

Conversation

A. スミスさんは先日の検査結果を聞くために診察室に入りました。会話を聞いて空所を埋めましょう。 DL 35 CD 35

● *In the Doctor's Office*

Doctor: Hello, Mr. Smith. Thank you for waiting. There were no problems with your (¹   ), but I have to explain your blood test results.

Mr. Smith: OK, Doctor. How was it?

Doctor: Well, you have high blood (²   ) levels, Mr. Smith. Your HbA1c value was 7.5. This should be (³   ).

Mr. Smith: What should I do, Doctor? Maybe I ate too many hamburgers and (⁴   ) fries.

Doctor: Aha... do you often feel thirsty?

Mr. Smith: Oh, yes, I do. Particularly during the (⁵   ). I feel thirsty and I go to the bathroom three times at night.

Doctor: Really? That's a lot.

B. スミスさんがたくさん食べた食べ物を、a〜cのイラストから選びましょう。

a 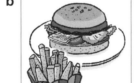   b   c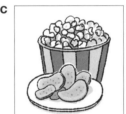

C. ペアになり、Doctor と Patient になったつもりでロールプレーをしましょう。日本語のセリフは英語に直して言ってみましょう。

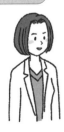 Doctor

You have high blood sugar levels. This should be lower.

What should I do, Doctor?

Patient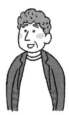

そうですね…、あなたはよく喉がかわきますか？

はい。特に夜間に。

More Expressions

A. 音声を聞き、空所を埋めましょう。　　　　　 DL 36　CD 36

> **1.** Your blood sugar (   ) are normal.
>
> **2.** I feel (   ) during the night.
>
> **3.** Your HbA1c was higher (   ) normal.
>
> **4.** What is the normal (   ) for HbA1c?
>
> **5.** Her medical (   ) is not serious.

B. 上の英文をヒントに、以下の日本語を英語に直しましょう。その後ペアになり、答えを確認しましょう。

1. 血糖値　　　　　　　(　　　　　　　　　　　　　　　　　　　　　　　　　　　　)
2. 喉がかわく　　　　　(　　　　　　　　　　　　　　　　　　　　　　　　　　　　)
3. 正常範囲　　　　　　(　　　　　　　　　　　　　　　　　　　　　　　　　　　　)
4. 病状　　　　　　　　(　　　　　　　　　　　　　　　　　　　　　　　　　　　　)
5. 標準より高い　　　　(　　　　　　　　　　　　　　　　　　　　　　　　　　　　)

🔊)) いくつ正解できましたか？

☐ 😊 5つ　　　　☐ 😐 3〜4つ　　　　☐ 😖 1〜2つ
Excellent　　　　　　　**Average**　　　　　　　**Poor**

Writing Challenge

以下の日本語を英語で書きましょう。

1. あなたのHbA1cは標準より高いです。

Your _____.

2. 私は夜に3、4回トイレに行きます。

_____ times a night.

3. 昨夜、私は喉がかわいていました。

I felt _____.

英文を読んで以下の問いに答えましょう。　　　 DL 37　 CD 37

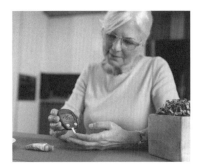

A high blood sugar level, also known as hyperglycemia, is a serious medical condition. Hyperglycemia is often confused with hypoglycemia, which is a low blood

5 sugar level. One way to remember the difference is to note that the word "low" shares a common sound "o" in the word hypoglycemia. Hyperglycemia is a common problem for people who suffer from type 1 or type 2 diabetes. It is important for people with diabetes

10 to recognize the symptoms of a high blood sugar level. This can include increased thirst, needing to urinate frequently and breath that smells fruity. A person's blood sugar level is known as the HbA1c level. A normal HbA1c level is considered to be between 4.6 and 6.2%. (120 words)

Note

urinate「排尿する」

1. What is another word for high blood sugar levels?

(a) Hypoglycemia

(b) Hyperglycemia

(c) Diabetes

2. Who is likely to suffer from the medical condition known as hyperglycemia?

(a) Only people with type 1 diabetes

(b) Only people with type 2 diabetes

(c) People with type 1 or type 2 diabetes

3. Which of the following can be symptoms of a high blood sugar level?

  (a) Increase in appetite

  (b) Increase in thirst

  (c) Increase in sleep

 Further Study

HbA1cとは過去1～2か月間の血糖値の平均で、HbA1cの正常な範囲は4.6%～6.2%とされていますが、4.6%～5.6%が良好な正常値と言われています。日本は、従来はこの厳しい値を正常値としていましたが、現在は4.6%～6.2%という世界の基準に合わせています。

世界的に糖尿病患者は増加傾向にあり、IDF（国際糖尿病連合）の予測では、2045年には世界で成人人口の12.2%にあたる7億8,300万人が糖尿病に苦しむとされています。以下はIDFが2021年に公開した、2045年までの糖尿病患者の増加率の予測を示した地図です。選択肢 a～ cの3つの地域を、増加率が高い順に並べ替えましょう。

Diabetes around the world 2021
Number of adults (20-79 years) with diabetes worldwide

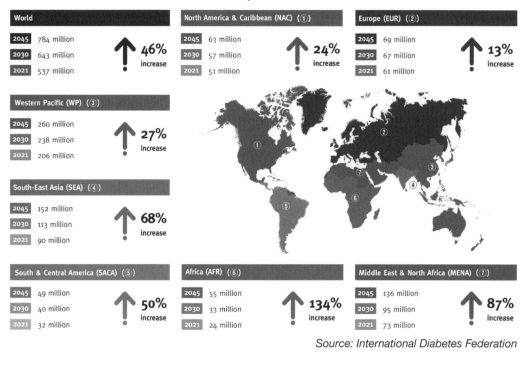

World	
2045 784 million	
2030 643 million	**46%** increase
2021 537 million	

North America & Caribbean (NAC) (①)	
2045 63 million	
2030 57 million	**24%** increase
2021 51 million	

Europe (EUR) (②)	
2045 69 million	
2030 67 million	**13%** increase
2021 61 million	

Western Pacific (WP) (③)	
2045 260 million	
2030 238 million	**27%** increase
2021 206 million	

South-East Asia (SEA) (④)	
2045 152 million	
2030 113 million	**68%** increase
2021 90 million	

South & Central America (SACA) (⑤)	
2045 49 million	
2030 40 million	**50%** increase
2021 32 million	

Africa (AFR) (⑥)	
2045 55 million	
2030 33 million	**134%** increase
2021 24 million	

Middle East & North Africa (MENA) (⑦)	
2045 136 million	
2030 95 million	**87%** increase
2021 73 million	

Source: International Diabetes Federation

[　　　→　　　→　　　]

a. ヨーロッパ　　b. 西太平洋　　c. 中東・北アフリカ

Unit 13

You Need to Control Your Diet

UNIT GOAL

☐ 患者に入院をすすめる
☐ 健康指導の表現を学ぶ

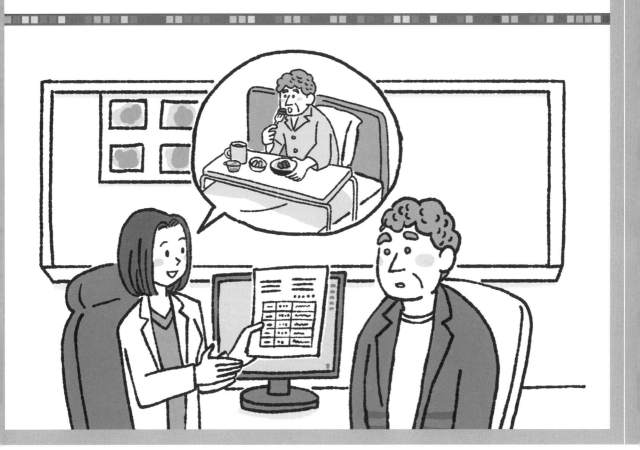

Key Words

以下の英語の意味を選択肢から記号で選び、書き入れましょう。

1. be strict with oneself （　） **a.** 食事を制限する

2. control one's diet （　） **b.** 自分に厳しくする

3. do one's best （　） **c.** 体重を管理する

4. control weight （　） **d.** 健康的な体重の減少

5. healthy weight loss （　） **e.** 最善を尽くす

Conversation

A. スミスさんは医師から説明を受けます。会話を聞いて空所を埋めましょう。

DL 38　　CD 38

● *In the Doctor's Office*

Doctor: Mr. Smith, I have to tell you that you have to be very strict with yourself when you need to (¹   ) your diet.

Mr. Smith: What do you (²   ), Doctor?

Doctor: Well, you had high blood sugar levels and your HbA1c value was 7.5. This value shows that your condition is (³   ).

Mr. Smith: What should I do, Doctor? I'll do my best to control my diet.

Doctor: Well, I understand, but diets will not be successful because controlling your weight through diets is not (⁴   ).

Mr. Smith: What should I do, Doctor?

Doctor: I'd like to (⁵   ) that you be hospitalized for healthy long-term weight loss.

B. 医師が説明したスミスさんの深刻な課題を、a〜cのイラストから選びましょう。

a

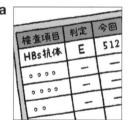

b

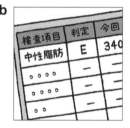

c

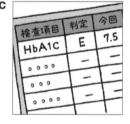

C. ペアになり、Patient と Doctor になったつもりでロールプレーをしましょう。日本語のセリフは英語に直して言ってみましょう。

Patient

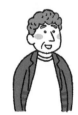

I'll do my best to control my diet.

I understand, but temporary diets will not be successful.

Doctor

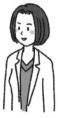

どうしたら良いでしょうか。

体重を減らすため、入院することをおすすめします。

More Expressions

A. 音声を聞き、空所を埋めましょう。 DL 39 CD 39

> **1.** Your condition is (　　　　　).
>
> **2.** I (　　　　　) that you be hospitalized.
>
> **3.** I'll do my (　　　　　) to lose weight.
>
> **4.** (　　　　　) diets can harm your health.
>
> **5.** His wife is very (　　　　　) about what he eats.

B. 上の英文をヒントに、以下の日本語を英語に直しましょう。その後ペアになり、答えを確認しましょう。

1. 入院する　　　　　　(　　　　　　　　　　　　　　　　　　　)

2. とても厳しい　　　　(　　　　　　　　　　　　　　　　　　　)

3. 体重を減らす努力をする　(　　　　　　　　　　　　　　　　　)

4. 一時的な食事制限　　(　　　　　　　　　　　　　　　　　　　)

5. 健康を害する　　　　(　　　　　　　　　　　　　　　　　　　)

 いくつ正解できましたか？

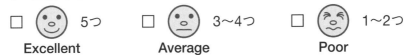

☐ 😊 5つ　　☐ 😐 3〜4つ　　☐ 😣 1〜2つ

Excellent　　　　**Average**　　　　**Poor**

Writing Challenge

以下の日本語を英語で書きましょう。

1. あなたは食事制限をする必要があります。

　You _____ .

2. 残念ながら、あなたの状態は深刻です。

　I'm afraid _____ .

3. あなたのHbA1cは正常の範囲内です。

　Your _____ .

Reading

英文を読んで以下の問いに答えましょう。　　　　　🎧 DL 40　💿 CD 40

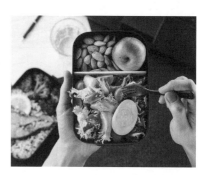

　　A person is likely to put on weight when the number of calories they eat is more than the number of calories they burn off during their normal daily activities and
5　exercise.　Controlling one's body weight through diet is not easy, but it is essential if we are to maintain a healthy body. Most medical institutions agree that temporary diets will only result in temporary loss of weight.　Fad diets that include low carbohydrate/high
10　protein diets and the popular 5:2 diet are not only difficult to maintain over a long period, they can also be unhealthy.　For healthy long-term weight loss, we should make small permanent changes to what we eat and drink and take regular daily exercise.　People who cannot make these changes by themselves may have to be hospitalized at some point.　　(135 words)

Notes

burn off...「～を燃焼する」　medical institution「医療機関」　fad diet「ファド・ダイエット（流行のダイエット法。特定の食品を排除するなどして短期間で減量することを目指すが、健康への悪影響が指摘されている）」
low carbohydrate/high protein diets「低糖質／高たんぱくダイエット」　5:2 diet「5:2ダイエット（1週間のうち2日を"断食日"として厳密なカロリー制限を行い、減量を目指す）」　permanent「永続的な」

1. According to most medical institutions, what is likely to happen to people who go on a fad diet?

(a) They will lose weight permanently.

(b) They will lose weight only temporarily.

(c) They will become healthier.

2. What is a negative aspect of fad diets like the 5:2 diet?

(a) They are easy to maintain over a long period of time.

(b) They are difficult to maintain over a long period of time.

(c) They help to maintain a healthy body weight.

3. What is recommended for people who want to maintain healthy long-term weight loss?

   (a) Make small temporary changes to what they eat and drink and take regular exercise

   (b) Make small permanent changes to what they eat and drink and take regular exercise

   (c) Make their own meals three times a day

Further Study

血糖値を下げるための食事療法にはさまざまな方法があります。まず主食（糖質）を減らすこと。次にたんぱく質を積極的にとり、野菜で食物繊維をしっかりとること。そして、食べる順番に気を付けることもよく言われていることです。
以下の写真の食品の中から、1. 糖質の多い食品、2. たんぱく質の多い食品、3. 食物繊維の多い食品の3つのカテゴリーに当てはまるものを、2つずつ選んでみましょう。

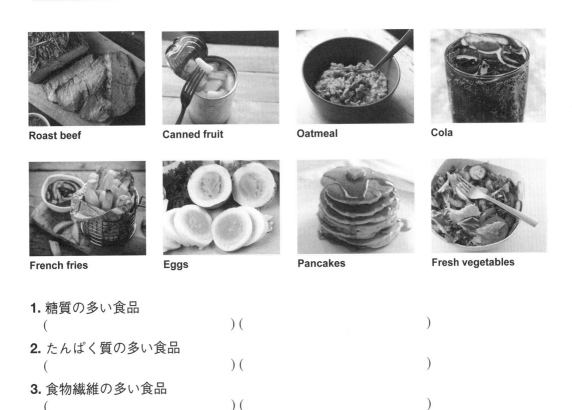

Roast beef   Canned fruit   Oatmeal   Cola

French fries   Eggs   Pancakes   Fresh vegetables

1. 糖質の多い食品
   (   ) (   )
2. たんぱく質の多い食品
   (   ) (   )
3. 食物繊維の多い食品
   (   ) (   )

Unit 14

You Need to Be Hospitalized

UNIT GOAL

☐ 入院前の説明をおこなう
☐ 入院に関する表現を学ぶ

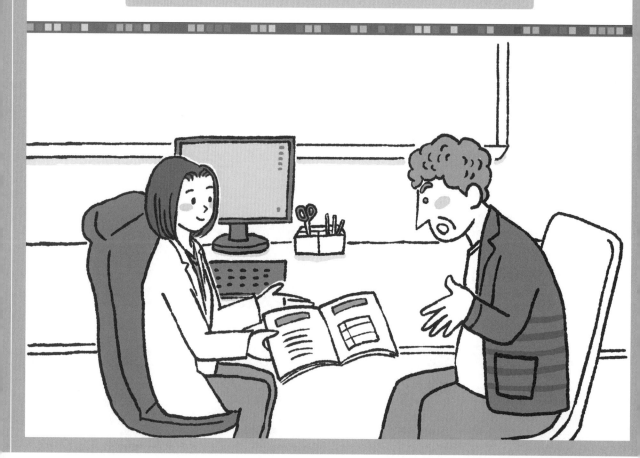

Key Words

以下の英語の意味を選択肢から記号で選び、書き入れましょう。

1. be hospitalized （　　） **a.** 少なくとも

2. at least （　　） **b.** 提案

3. go down （　　） **c.** 入院する

4. suggestion （　　） **d.** 下がる

5. handbook （　　） **e.** 案内書

Conversation

A. スミスさんは入院についての説明を受けます。会話を聞いて空所を埋めましょう。

DL 41 CD 41

● *In the Doctor's Office*

Doctor: I recommend that you be hospitalized because it's difficult to control your (¹   ) by yourself.

Mr. Smith: How long should I be hospitalized, Doctor?

Doctor: You should be hospitalized for at least a month.

Mr. Smith: For a month? (²   ) a long time?

Doctor: Of course. If you're hospitalized for a month, your blood sugar (³   ) will go down.

Mr. Smith: I understand. I'll follow your suggestion.

Doctor: Here is a handbook for hospitalization. It (⁴   ) information such as what to bring for your hospital stay.

Mr. Smith: OK. I'll have a look at it with my (⁵   ).

B. スミスさんは病院から帰宅後に何をすると言っていますか。a〜cのイラストから選びましょう。

a 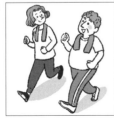　　b 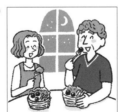　　c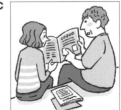

C. ペアになり、PatientとDoctorになったつもりでロールプレーをしましょう。日本語のセリフは英語に直して言ってみましょう。

Patient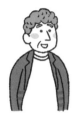

How long should I be hospitalized, doctor?

You should be hospitalized for at least a month.

Doctor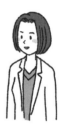

1か月間？そんなに長い間ですか？

もちろんです。1か月間入院すれば、あなたの血糖値は下がるでしょう。

More Expressions

A. 音声を聞き、空所を埋めましょう。　　　　　 DL 42　　CD 42

> **1.** How long should I be (　　　　　　)?
>
> **2.** What should I bring for my hospital (　　　　　　)?
>
> **3.** Please sign the necessary (　　　　　) before hospitalization.
>
> **4.** No visitors are (　　　　　) due to the COVID-19 pandemic.
>
> **5.** Where can I (　　　　　) a discharge certificate?

B. 上の英文をヒントに、以下の日本語を英語に直しましょう。

1. 入院する　　　　　(　　　　　　　　　　　　　　　　　　　　)

2. 必要書類　　　　　(　　　　　　　　　　　　　　　　　　　　)

3. 新型コロナのため　(　　　　　　　　　　　　　　　　　　　　)

4. 退院証明書　　　　(　　　　　　　　　　　　　　　　　　　　)

 いくつ正解できましたか？

☐ 😊 4つ　　　　☐ 😐 2〜3つ　　　☐ 😣 1つ
Excellent　　　　　　Average　　　　　　Poor

Writing Challenge

以下の日本語を英語で書きましょう。

1. 食事管理を自分でするのは難しいです。

It is _____ by yourself.

2. あなたの血糖値は2週間で下がるでしょう。

Your blood sugar level _____.

3. 少なくとも2週間の入院が必要です。

You should _____.

英文を読んで以下の問いに答えましょう。 DL 43 CD 43

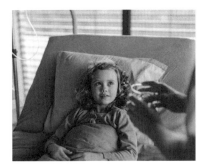

When a patient is admitted to a hospital, it is simply a medical way of saying a patient is entering a hospital to receive medical treatment over an 5 extended period of time. It can be for a couple of days, weeks, months, and in the worst cases, years. When the medical treatment is complete, the patient is discharged, which means that they leave the hospital to go home. An extended stay in a hospital can be a 10 stressful time for an adult patient, but it is particularly stressful for young children. A nurse can help reduce a patient's stress in a number of ways. One way is speaking to the patient in a friendly and reassuring voice. Also, it is important to explain the hospital procedures in a way they are likely to understand, avoiding any unnecessary medical language. (139 words)

Notes

over an extended period of time「長期間にわたって」　reassuring「安心させるような」

1. What does the term "admitted to a hospital" mean?

(a) A patient is entering a hospital to receive medical treatment over an extended period of time.

(b) A patient is entering a hospital after medical treatment is complete.

(c) A patient is visiting the hospital for the first time.

2. What does the term "discharged from a hospital" mean?

(a) A patient is entering a hospital to receive medical treatment over an extended period of time.

(b) A patient is leaving a hospital after medical treatment is complete.

(c) A patient does not want to receive medical treatment over an extended period of time.

3. What should nurses avoid when explaining hospital procedures to patients?

   (a) Speaking in a friendly and reassuring voice

   (b) Speaking slowly

   (c) Using unnecessary medical language

Further Study

入院期間中、患者は不安や孤独を感じやすいものです。家族や友人にお見舞いに来てもらい、息抜きをしたいと願う患者も少なくないでしょう。その場合には、病院で定められている面会のルールをよく確認しておきましょう。
以下の面会ルールについて、下の１〜３の質問に答えましょう。

HOSPITAL RULES AND REGULATIONS

<u>To visitors:</u>

   ✓ Visitors are limited to two per patient at one time.
   ✓ Maintain low voice tones in all areas of the hospital.
   ✓ Adhere to visiting hours.
   ✓ Restrict calls to patient rooms after 9 p.m.
   ✓ Avoid waiting in hallways in patient care areas.

---

1. １人の患者につき１度に面会できるのは何人までですか。（　　　　　　　　）

2. 病院内の全てのエリアで気をつけることは何ですか。（　　　　　　　　　　）

3. 入院患者の部屋に電話できるのは何時までですか。（　　　　　　　）

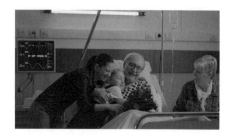

Unit 15
Keep on Walking for Exercise

UNIT GOAL

- ☐ 退院後のアドバイスをおこなう
- ☐ 健康維持に関する表現を学ぶ

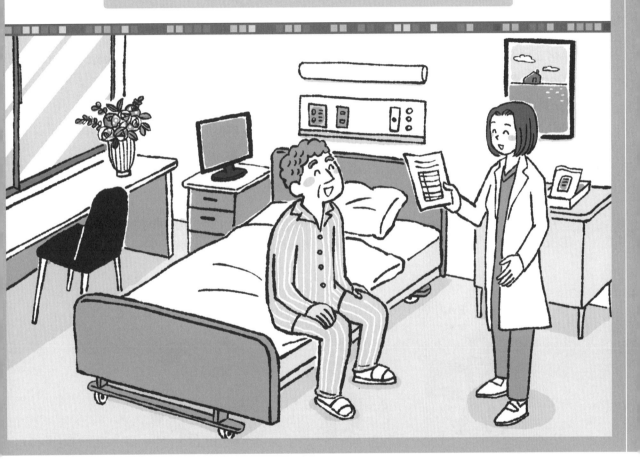

Key Words

以下の英語の意味を選択肢から記号で選び、書き入れましょう。

1. Time flies.	( )	**a.** 退院する
2. leave the hospital	( )	**b.** 近い将来
3. medical check-up	( )	**c.** 光陰矢の如し
4. exercise	( )	**d.** 運動
5. in the near future	( )	**e.** 健康診断

Conversation

A. 入院後 1 か月が経過し、スミスさんは医師から説明を受けます。会話を聞いて空所を埋めましょう。 DL 44　CD 44

● *In the Patient's Room*

Doctor: It has been a (¹   ) since you were hospitalized.

Mr. Smith: Time flies. I heard that my HbA1c level was 6.2 this time.

Doctor: That's right. It is within the normal range, Mr. Smith.

Mr. Smith: Very (²   ) to hear that. When can I leave the hospital?

Doctor: The day after tomorrow. You need to have a medical (³   )
before you leave.

Mr. Smith: I heard about that, Doctor. I'm going to start walking for exercise in
the near future.

Doctor: That's a good idea, Mr. Smith. (⁴   ) on walking for exercise
for 30 to 40 minutes every day.

Mr. Smith: I know some exercise is necessary for lowering my blood sugar level.

Doctor: Yes, (⁵   ). I've also been walking for exercise for about
10 years.

B. 医師はスミスさんに何をすすめていますか。a ～ c のイラストから選びましょう。

a
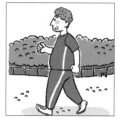
b
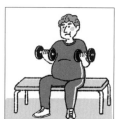
c
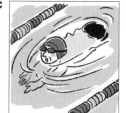

C. ペアになり、Patient と Doctor になったつもりでロールプレーをしましょう。日本語のセリフは英語に直して言ってみましょう。

Patient
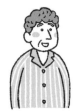

I heard that I can leave the hospital the day after tomorrow.

Yes, but you need to have a medical check-up before you leave.

Doctor
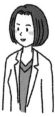

聞いています。
近いうちに、ウォーキングの運動を始める予定です。

それは
いい考えですね！

More Expressions

A. 音声を聞き、空所を埋めましょう。 DL 45 CD 45

> 1. I'm very ( ) to hear my test results.
>
> 2. I'm ( ) the hospital tomorrow.
>
> 3. You need to have a medical ( ) in the morning.
>
> 4. Work out for at ( ) 30 minutes every day.
>
> 5. I'll keep ( ) playing tennis after I graduate from school.

B. 上の英文をヒントに、以下の日本語を英語に直しましょう。その後ペアになり、答えを確認しましょう。

1. 30分間運動する　　　　　(　　　　　　　　　　　　　　　　　　　　　　)
2. 検査結果を聞く　　　　　(　　　　　　　　　　　　　　　　　　　　　　)
3. 健康診断を受ける　　　　(　　　　　　　　　　　　　　　　　　　　　　)
4. テニスを続ける　　　　　(　　　　　　　　　　　　　　　　　　　　　　)
5. 退院する　　　　　　　　(　　　　　　　　　　　　　　　　　　　　　　)

 いくつ正解できましたか？

 5つ　　　 3〜4つ　　　 1〜2つ

　　Excellent　　　　　　　**Average**　　　　　　　**Poor**

Writing Challenge

以下の日本語を英語で書きましょう。

1. あなたは明後日退院することができます。

_____ the day after tomorrow.

2. 毎日、最低1時間は運動しましょう。

_____ every day.

3. 10年以上毎朝ウォーキングの運動を行っています。

I've been _____ .

Reading

英文を読んで以下の問いに答えましょう。

 DL 46 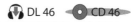 CD 46

Regular exercise is of great benefit in maintaining a healthy body. However, an overweight person who is thinking about starting an exercise program should first have a medical check-up. After the check-up, a doctor will be able to recommend an exercise routine that best fits their condition. Most medical practitioners agree that an overweight person should begin with very moderate exercise at first, slowly building up the number and extent of any exercises. A popular exercise routine with beginners is known as "Couch to 5K." This routine begins with running very slowly for about 10 minutes a day, and very slowly increasing the distance and time over a period of about nine weeks. The aim of this course is to be able to run 5 kilometers in about 30 minutes.

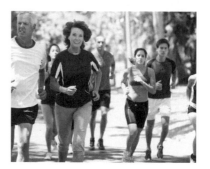

(130 words)

Notes

be of great benefit「非常に有益である」   medical practitioner「医師」

1. What will a doctor be able to recommend to a patient after a medical check-up?

(a) An exercise routine best suited to their body condition

(b) An exercise routine best suited to promote lean muscle growth

(c) An exercise routine best suited to a patient's sporting aims

2. When an overweight person starts an exercise routine, what do most medical practitioners agree on?

(a) The routine should be long and a little painful.

(b) The routine should begin with very moderate exercise.

(c) The routine should be accompanied by a large increase in food intake.

3. What is the aim of the routine known as "Couch to 5K?"

   (a) To be able to run 5 kilometers in 10 minutes

   (b) To be able to run 5 kilometers in 20 minutes

   (c) To be able to run 5 kilometers in 30 minutes

Further Study

Readingで紹介されていたCouch to 5Kというランニングのためのプログラムは、1996年にジョシュ・クラークという男性によって開発されました。元々、彼はランニングを辛く苦しいものだと思っていましたが、失恋の悲しみを忘れるためにランニングを始めたところ、徐々に走ることが快感になっていきました。こうして彼は多くの人と、「誰にでもできる」ランニングのトレーニングをシェアしたいと思ったのでした。

今ではCouch to 5Kのメソッドを実践できるアプリが人気で、実際に人々が集まってランニングトレーニングを行うイベントも開催されるまでになりました。以下は、そうしたイベントの告知ポスターです。1～3の質問に答えましょう。

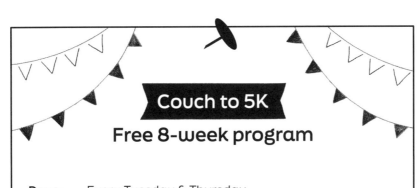

Couch to 5K
Free 8-week program

Days: Every Tuesday & Thursday
            October 15th through December 10th
Time: 6pm – 7pm
Venue: Johnson Memorial Park
Bring: water, running shoes and layers

The program is for absolute beginners.
Get ready to run with the help of our qualified coaches!

Please contact us at **running@exciting.com** to register.

1. プログラムの参加費はいくらですか。(　　　　　　　　　　)

2. 持ち物は何ですか。(　　　　　　　　　　　　　　　　)

3. 初心者には誰が教えてくれますか。(　　　　　　　　　)

✛ Useful Expressions ✛

医療の現場でよく使われる表現を一覧にしました。
声に出して発音し、習得しましょう。

◆＝本編に登場した表現　◇＝それ以外の表現

📋 1. 患者の受付をする・案内する

◆ May I help you? — どうなさいましたか。

◆ Is this your first visit to this hospital? — この病院に来るのは初めてですか。

◇ Do you have an appointment? — 予約を取っていますか。

◆ Please go to the Registration Desk. — 登録カウンターへ行ってください。

◆ May I have your name and date of birth? — お名前と生年月日を教えてください。

◆ May I ask your marital status? — ご結婚されていますか。

◆ Do you have an insurance card? — 保険証をお持ちですか。

◇ Please fill in [out] this registration form. — この登録票に記入してください。

◆ Your registration card is ready. — 診察券が準備できました。

◇ Please wait here. A nurse will call your name/number.
ここでお待ちください。看護師がお名前／番号をお呼びします。

◆ Your doctor is coming soon to see you. — 医師がすぐに診察に来ます。

◆ Please have a seat. — どうぞお座りください。

◆ What department do you want to visit? — どの診療科を受診されますか。

◇ I'll show you the way to the Blood Test Room. — 採血室への行き方をご案内します。

◇ Internal Medicine is on the second floor next to Surgery.
内科は２階、外科の隣にあります。

🩺 2. 症状について聞く・話す

◆ What are your symptoms? — どのような症状ですか。

◆ What seems to be your problem? — 何が問題と思われますか。

◆ How are you feeling today? — 今日のご気分はいかがですか。

◇ How can I help? — どうされましたか。

◆ How long have you been coughing? — どのくらいせきが続いていますか。

◇ How long have you been experiencing...? — どのくらい〜が続いていますか。

◆ Did you check your temperature? — 体温を測りましたか。

77

◆ What kind of pain is it?	どのような痛みですか。
◇ Does it hurt when I touch...?	～を触ると痛いですか。
◆ I have a fever.	熱があります。
◆ I feel dizzy.	めまいがします。
◆ I feel nauseous.	吐き気がします。
◆ I have a headache.	頭痛がします。
◆ My eyes are itchy and watery.	目がかゆく、涙目になります。
◆ I have a runny nose.	鼻水が出ています。
◆ I sneeze a lot and have a stuffy nose.	くしゃみがたくさん出て、鼻がつまります。
◆ Currently, I have a slight fever.	現在、微熱があります。
◆ I don't feel good lately.	最近、具合が悪いです。
◇ I have been coughing for a while.	しばらくせきが続いています。
◇ I have a dry cough.	空ぜきが出ます。
◇ I have slight chills.	少し寒気がします。
◇ I think I may have a cold.	風邪をひいているかもしれません。
◆ I feel pain in my back.	背中に痛みがあります。
◆ It's a dull pain and it is constant.	鈍い痛みで、持続的です。
◇ The pain is getting worse day by day.	痛みが日に日にひどくなっています。
◇ I have chronic headaches.	慢性的な頭痛があります。
◇ I have a stinging pain in my stomach.	腹部がちくちく痛みます。
◇ I have a sore throat.	喉が痛いです。
◇ My bones ache.	骨が痛いです。

3. 検査する・診察する

◆ Let's check your temperature.	検温しましょう。
◆ Let's check your pulse and blood pressure.	脈と血圧を測りましょう。
◆ Let's check your daily activities.	生活習慣を見てみましょう。
◇ Let's check your weight and height.	体重と身長を測りましょう。
◇ Do you have a health check every year?	毎年健康診断を受けていますか。
◇ Please lie on the bed.	ベッドに横になってください。
◇ Please put your arm on this table.	腕をこのテーブルに置いてください。
◇ Please take a deep breath.	大きく深呼吸してください。

◇ You'll have a blood test tomorrow. 明日、血液検査をします。

◇ We offer a COVID-19 PCR test. PCR 検査を受けることができます。

◇ Would you like to have a gastroscopy? 胃カメラ検査をご希望ですか。

◇ We may need to run a few tests. いくつか検査が必要です。

◇ Let us take X-rays. レントゲンを撮らせてください。

◇ When can I take those tests? それらの検査はいつ受けられますか。

◇ When will you have the test results? 検査結果はいつ出ますか。

◆ Your pulse was 70; no problem at all. 脈は 70 で、まったく問題ありません。

◆ Your blood pressure is 110 over 80. 血圧は上が 110, 下が 80 です。

◆ You have high/low blood pressure. 高血圧／低血圧です。

◆ You have high blood sugar levels. 血糖値が高いです。

◆ Your HbA1c value was 7.5. HbA1c の値が 7.5 です。

◆ This should be lower. この値を下げなくてはなりません。

◆ I think you're suffering from hay fever. 花粉症のようですね。

◇ You have tested positive/negative. 検査結果は陽性／陰性でした。

◇ You are infected with COVID-19. 新型コロナウイルスに感染しています。

◆ Some inflammations were found in your stomach. 胃に炎症が見つかりました。

◆ This value shows that your condition is serious. この数値は深刻な状態を示しています。

◇ You have to be strict with what you eat. 食事制限が必要です。

◇ Do you have any questions? 何か質問はありますか。

◇ Take care. お大事にしてください。

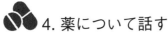 4. 薬について話す

◇ Let me take your prescription. 処方箋をお預かりします。

◇ Do you have your medicine notebook? お薬手帳をお持ちですか。

◇ Your prescription will be ready in 10 minutes. お薬は 10 分でご用意できます。

◇ Are you being treated for any disease? 現在何らかの病気の治療中ですか。

◇ Are you pregnant or breastfeeding? 妊娠中または授乳中ですか。

◇ Do you have any allergies to medications? 薬にアレルギーはありますか。

◇ Would you prefer the generic brand? ジェネリック医薬品をご希望ですか。

◆ Your medicine is ready.　　　　　　　　　　　お薬が準備できました。

◆ These tablets are antibiotics.　　　　　　　　これらの錠剤は抗生物質です。

◆ They help ease coughing.　　　　　　　　　　せきを和らげます。

◆ We'll prescribe you medicine: antihistamines.　抗ヒスタミンという薬を処方します。

◆ These medicines help ease allergy symptoms.　この薬はアレルギー症状を緩和します。

◇ This stops diarrhea.　　　　　　　　　　　　これは下痢止めです。

◆ Take one tablet three times after meals.　　　毎食後3回1錠飲んでください。

◆ Take this medicine as needed.　　　　　　　この薬を必要に応じて飲んでください。

◇ Take this with plenty of water.　　　　　　　たっぷりの水で飲んでください。

◇ Dissolve this in water before drinking.　　　　飲む前に水に溶かしてください。

◆ You can take pain reliever when you have a fever.　発熱時は解熱剤を飲んでもよいです。

◇ Take two capsules every four hours.　　　　　4時間ごとに2カプセル飲んでください。

◇ Let... hours pass between doses.　　　　　　服用後〜時間あけてください。

◇ This is enough medicine for... days.　　　　　〜日分の薬です。

◇ Store the medicine in a cool, dry place.　　　薬は涼しく乾燥した場所に保管してください。

5. 入退院について話す

◆ I recommend that you be hospitalized.　　　　入院することをおすすめします。

◇ You need to be admitted.　　　　　　　　　　入院が必要です。

◇ You don't have to be admitted; just take medications for a month.

　　　　　　　　　　入院の必要はありません。1か月間の服薬治療で十分です。

◆ How long should I be hospitalized?　　　　　どのくらいの期間入院が必要ですか。

◆ You should be hospitalized for at least a month.　最低1か月間入院が必要です。

◆ Here is a handbook for hospitalization.　　　こちらが入院の案内書です。

◆ Please sign the necessary documents before hospitalization.

　　　　　　　　　　入院前に、必要書類に署名してください。

◇ Visiting hours are 10 a.m. to 6 p.m.　　　　面会時間は午前10時〜午後6時です。

◆ No visitors are allowed due to the COVID-19 pandemic.

　　　　　　　　　　新型コロナウイルス対策のため、面会禁止です。

◆ When can I leave the hospital?　　　　　　　いつ退院できますか。

◆ You need to have a medical check-up before you leave.

　　　　　　　　　　退院前に検診を受ける必要があります。

◇ Here is your discharge certificate.　　　　　こちらが退院証明書です。

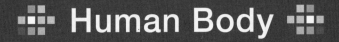

Human Body

医療の現場で役に立つ身体の部位の名称を掲載しました。
それぞれの図を見ながらしっかり覚えましょう。

Head（頭部）

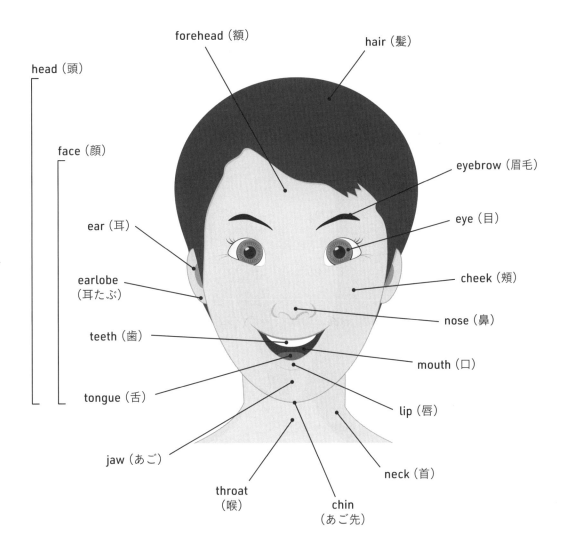

forehead（額）

hair（髪）

head（頭）

face（顔）

eyebrow（眉毛）

eye（目）

ear（耳）

earlobe
（耳たぶ）

cheek（頬）

nose（鼻）

teeth（歯）

mouth（口）

tongue（舌）

lip（唇）

jaw（あご）

neck（首）

throat
（喉）

chin
（あご先）

Body Parts（身体の部位）

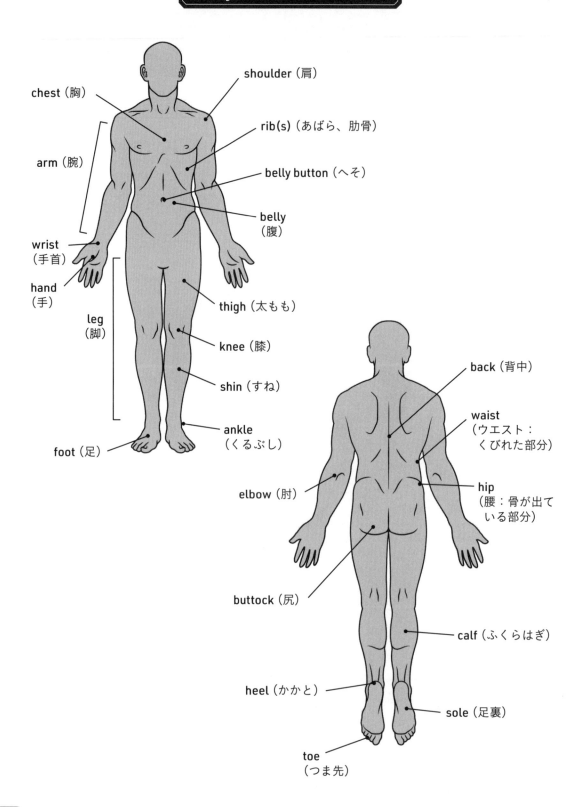

chest（胸）

shoulder（肩）

rib(s)（あばら、肋骨）

arm（腕）

belly button（へそ）

belly（腹）

wrist（手首）

hand（手）

thigh（太もも）

leg（脚）

knee（膝）

shin（すね）

ankle（くるぶし）

foot（足）

back（背中）

waist（ウエスト：くびれた部分）

hip（腰：骨が出ている部分）

elbow（肘）

buttock（尻）

calf（ふくらはぎ）

heel（かかと）

sole（足裏）

toe（つま先）

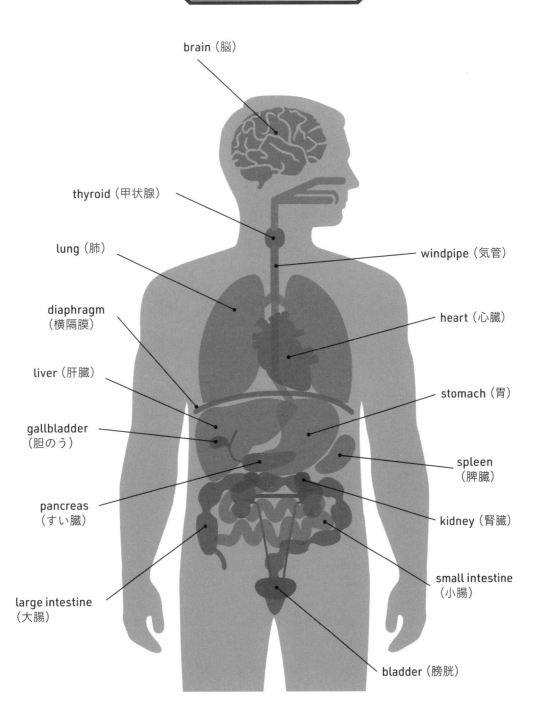

brain（脳）

thyroid（甲状腺）

lung（肺）

diaphragm
（横隔膜）

liver（肝臓）

gallbladder
（胆のう）

pancreas
（すい臓）

large intestine
（大腸）

windpipe（気管）

heart（心臓）

stomach（胃）

spleen
（脾臓）

kidney（腎臓）

small intestine
（小腸）

bladder（膀胱）

本書にはCD（別売）があります

Check-Up!
Basic English for Nursing
基礎から学ぶ やさしい看護英語

| 2023年1月20日　初版第1刷発行 |
| 2024年2月20日　初版第3刷発行 |

| 著　者 | 樋 口 晶 彦 |
| | John Tremarco |

| 発行者 | 福 岡 正 人 |
| 発行所 | 株式会社　金 星 堂 |

（〒101-0051）　東京都千代田区神田神保町 3-21
Tel　（03）3263-3828（営業部）
　　　（03）3263-3997（編集部）
Fax　（03）3263-0716
https://www.kinsei-do.co.jp

編集担当　戸田浩平・蔦原美智　　　　　　　　　Printed in Japan
印刷所／日新印刷株式会社　製本所／松島製本
本書の無断複製・複写は著作権法上での例外を除き禁じられています。本書を代
行業者等の第三者に依頼してスキャンやデジタル化することは、たとえ個人や家
庭内での利用であっても認められておりません。
落丁・乱丁本はお取り替えいたします。

ISBN978-4-7647-4184-3　　C1082